MICROBIOLOGY FOR NURSES

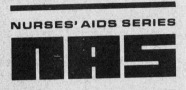

NURSES' AIDS SERIES

Microbiology for Nurses

Sixth Edition

3719398

616.01024613.

Margaret J. Parker
SRN

Nursing Administration (Hospital) Certificate;
Formerly Nurse Epidemiologist,
The Department of Community Medicine,
The Middlesex Hospital Medical School, London

Vivien A. Stucke
SRN
Certificate in Oncology Nursing; Formerly Nursing Officer,
Infection Control, The Middlesex Hospital, London

Foreword by the late

R.E.M. Thompson
MB, BS, FRCPath
Consultant Bacteriologist, The Middlesex Hospital, London.
Reader in Bacteriology, The Middlesex Hospital Medical School,
London

BAILLIÈRE TINDALL
LONDON

Published by BAILLIÈRE TINDALL,
a division of Cassell Ltd,
Greycoat House, 10 Greycoat Place,
London SW1P 1SB

an affiliate of
Macmillan Publishing Co. Inc.
New York

First published as *Bacteriology for Nurses* 1959
Fifth edition 1978
   Reprinted 1979, 1980
Sixth edition 1982

ISBN 0 7020 0924 5

Educational Low-priced Book Series Editions 1969, 1972, 1978
Spanish edition (CECSA, Mexico) 1972

British Library Cataloguing in Publication Data
Parker, Margaret J.
   Microbiology for nurses.—6th ed.—(Nurses' aids series)
   1. Medical microbiology
   I. Title II. Stucke, Vivien A. III. Series
   616'.01'024613 QR46

   ISBN 0–7020–0924–5

Printed in Great Britain by Spottiswoode Ballantyne,
Colchester, Essex

Photoset by Enset Ltd, Midsomer Norton, Bath, Avon

Contents

Foreword

I feel honoured to be asked to write the foreword to the sixth edition of this useful book. The importance of nurses in the control and prevention of infection in hospitals has been more and more recognized in recent years so that nowadays any general hospital that does not have a nurse as part of the infection control team could be looked on as rather backward in this field.

One of the major functions of such a nurse is education in anti-infection measures of nurses, lay staff of all grades and often, be it said, medical staff. This book provides a simple, easily understood résumé of medical microbiology and the functioning of the laboratory. It is written in simple language from the viewpoint of a general hospital and is therefore valuable to those undertaking general nurse training.

June 1981   R.E.M. Thompson

Preface

An understanding of microbiology is essential for all nurses if they are to work safely in both hospital and community environments, to maintain asepsis and prevent the spread of infection. This book has always been aimed at helping both learners and qualified nurses in many situations to appreciate the importance of microbiology, and this edition is intended to further that aim. I hope that the additional material will both keep nurses abreast of new knowledge, and emphasize their practical role in preventing and controlling infection in hospitals and elsewhere.

Additions have been made to most chapters, and one new chapter included. In particular, the chapter on immunity has been expanded to include the exciting new developments in immunology with special reference to the complement system which has a major role in destruction of infecting organisms, information on the different types of antibody and other advances. The chapters on pathogenic bacteria and on viruses contain information now available on organisms such as Legionella and Marburg virus. Some reorganization has been made in the chapters on infection and sterilization and disinfection, mostly in connection with the expanded coverage of applied microbiology.

The chapter on that subject now also includes information about infection control teams, and nurses in particular, as their role is increasingly understood and appreciated, and the relevance of anti-infection measures in the community is also discussed. Further applied microbiology chapters on the principles of isolation have been included with particular emphasis on practical guidance and a humane, patient-orientated approach to the problems associated with isolating people with infections, reinforced by the necessary understanding of why isolation is needed.

All these alterations and additions are intended to make the book of even more practical help to the nurse working in hospital and community while maintaining sufficiently detailed information to satisfy a nurse's thirst for information in depth. This intention has clearly been behind the last two editions of this book by Miss M.J. Parker which I am delighted to have been asked to follow, and hope readers will find this a worthy successor.

I am much indebted to three members of the School of Pathology of the Middlesex Hospital Medical School for help and advice on the text. Dr Graham Rook's help with the last edition's new chapter on immunity was very well received and his contribution this time will, I am sure, be equally helpful. Dr D.M.S. Dane has again provided new photographic material for the chapter on viruses and a great deal of time and interest in updating the material in that chapter. Dr R.E.M. Thompson has again written the foreword and has been invaluable in helping me to prepare this new edition of a book to which he has contributed so much over the last ten years. It is largely due to his teaching and patience that I have gained the interest and knowledge of microbiology and infection control which enabled me to prepare this edition.

I gratefully acknowledge permission to reproduce illustrations as follows: Mark Hayes for *The great germ fighters—soap and water* and *All things must pass—even isolation!;* Figs. 1, 2 and 3 from original photographs in the Wellcome Institute of the History of Medicine, by courtesy of the Wellcome Trustees; Fig. 4 from Dr P.N. Cardew,

Fig. 30 from Hazen, E.L. and Curtis Read, F. Laboratory Identification of Pathogenic Fungi Simplified, 2nd edn, 1960 by courtesy of Charles C. Thomas, Springfield, Illinois; and Fig. 47 from P.D. Whitehead. Finally, the publication *Isolation Techniques for Use in Hospitals* by the US Department of Health, Education and Welfare, from which the isolation categories were developed.

Sadly, since completion of this edition, Dr R.E.M. Thompson has died. His contribution to the fields of microbiology and infection control cannot be overstated. The time which he spent passing on this expertise has been of value to the many nurses who have benefited from his ability to explain complex technical concepts in simple, understandable terms. He will be greatly missed.

March 1982   Vivien A. Stucke

1 Introduction

Microbiology, the study of micro-organisms including bacteria, viruses, rickettsiae, fungi and yeasts, may seem a mainly academic subject to the student nurse, and of limited value in the care of her patients. However, these organisms with very diverse patterns of behaviour and environmental preferences vary in activity from those positively benefiting man, through the majority of harmless organisms to those which can cause disease and even death. An understanding of the way in which they work is essential for a nurse to apply the principles of asepsis and those involved in the control of infection. When it is realized that 5–10% of hospital patients acquire some form of infection, nurses will wish to do their utmost to help the patient recover or even prevent the situation arising, by applying their microbiological knowledge in the practical skills designed to prevent or control infection.

The principles of personal, hospital and community hygiene are based on an understanding of microbiology. It touches life at every point, from such personal matters as bathing, ventilating a bedroom, and eating habits, to comprehensive public services such as the supply of water, drainage and building works, or the activities of port sanitary authorities. Microbiological interest stretches from the kitchen where the housewife prepares food for the freezer, via the baby whose existence may be threatened by a dirty feeding bottle or teat, to the involved preparations for feeding the space explorer whose life may depend upon the preservation of his food supplies. The effects of poor hygiene in the home are unpleasant, in a hospital they can be disastrous. Unwashed hands or a dirty, fly-ridden kitchen lead to contamination of food and subsequently to diarrhoea and vomiting in the family; a shared towel in the bathroom may spread impetigo. In hospital, because of the lowered resistance of sick patients and the greater concentration of pathogenic organisms, faulty hygiene is more likely to cause serious outbreaks of infection spreading rapidly among patients, staff and even to the community.

Infection is a hazard to any patient; it prolongs treatment in hospital, with pain or discomfort, loss of working time and income, and worry and inconvenience for the relatives. The economic and social effects on the hospital and the community are considerable, ranging from increased drug and dressing bills, lowered bed occupancy rates and disruption of admission arrangements, to litigation. The emergence of drug-resistant strains of bacteria may be increased by the extensive use of antibiotics in the treatment of the victims. Those nursed at home will be exposed to some of the problems but are generally less liable to secondary infection and when it occurs are less likely to be attacked by infecting organisms that are particularly resistant to antibiotics.

To nurses more than to most sections of the community is given both the knowledge and the opportunity of practising what has been learnt in this field. This book has been written to further an earnest hope that the practice of nursing will be based in the future on an even more conscientious application of sound microbiological knowledge and principles. Since it has been written for student nurses it has been applied mainly to the hospital field. Nevertheless, the principles it embodies are of the greatest importance in the home, in the community and in every sphere of nursing experience.

2 The History of Microbiology

The history of microbiology is short. Modern ideas on the subject can be said to have started in 1546 when Fracastoro was the first to suggest that infection is composed of minute, insensible particles and is spread by means of them. He noted that the infection was the same for 'he who received as for he who had given' the infection. This was a great advance, recognizing as it did the transmission of disease. Nevertheless, although contagion was generally recognized in some diseases, as in the plague and in syphilis, in others it was still missed.

For centuries all races used the products of bacterial growth and fermentation without realizing the implications of the changes or the processes involved. In fact, the relationship between fermentation and infectious disease was not suspected until two centuries after bacteria were first seen by Antonius van Leeuwenhoek in 1676, using primitive microscopes of his own design and making.

In 1776 Spallanzani first cultivated bacteria in sterilized media, with and without air. He failed, however, to realize the importance of this and either was unaware of Fracastoro's work or failed to relate it to his own.

While this work was being carried on by the scientists, the causation of infectious disease was being investigated empirically by the clinicians of the day. In 1767 John Hunter, investigating the cause of syphilis, experimentally infected himself. Unfortunately, he induced a mixed infection of gonorrhoea and syphilis and his results were, because of this, confused. In 1796 Jenner, a pupil of

Hunter, introduced vaccination, making use of the practical observation that those who had cowpox were immune or partially immune to smallpox.

In 1847 Semmelweiss, a Viennese obstetrician, realized that puerperal fever was transmitted from one patient to another on the hands of the attendants. He showed conclusively that infection could be greatly reduced by hand-washing and the use of a mild antiseptic (chlorinated lime) on the skin. This discovery is the foundation stone of all modern aseptic techniques in use in hospitals.

A few years later in 1854 Dr John Snow demonstrated that cholera was transmitted through drinking water by showing the geographical relationship of the cases to the Broad Street pump in London and then stopping the outbreak by removing the pump handle.

Improvements in the microscope led to special diseases being associated with certain organisms of characteristic morphology. Davaine in 1850 saw what he called minute 'infusoria' in the blood of sheep dead from anthrax and he

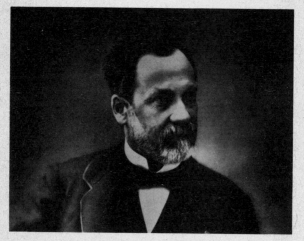

Fig. 1. Louis Pasteur (1822–1895).

was able to transmit the disease by inoculation of greatly diluted blood.

The techniques of modern microbiology were largely initiated and enormously developed by Pasteur, Lister and Koch. Pasteur, a pure chemist, became interested through investigation of industrial fermentation problems. He demonstrated that alcoholic fermentation was brought about by specific bacterial enzymes, and gave a logical explanation for a process which had been carried on for hundreds of years.

Lister followed up Pasteur's work on fermentation and carried out experiments to test the deduction that if fermentation of sugar and starch was due to bacterial action, sepsis and putrefaction of proteins were due to a similar cause. He therefore attempted to prevent bacterial invasion of operation wounds and injuries and the many forms of sepsis which resulted in suppuration, hospital gangrene and septicaemia. He used phenol to destroy germs and prevent them gaining a foothold in wounds. He

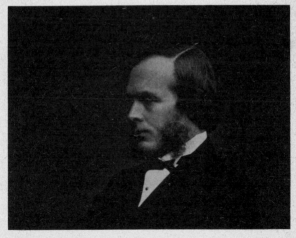

Fig. 2. Lord Lister (1827–1912).

published the successful results of his work in 1867, though it was many years before many of his sceptical colleagues accepted his teaching. By applying carbolic putty to cases of compound fracture, he was able to save limbs which would previously have been amputated because of the risk of a fatal result from gangrene or septicaemia. In the course of his experiments he devised a technique for obtaining pure cultures originating from a single organism, the first man to do so.

While Pasteur was working in France and Lister in England, Koch in Germany was developing the bacteriological techniques which form the basis of modern diagnostic bacteriology. Today it is relatively simple to identify an unknown organism. The necessary tests have been laid down and are simply a matter of applying routine knowledge, but in 1870 Koch had no such rules to help him and new disciplines had to be worked out. Koch isolated the bacillus of anthrax, the first pathogenic organism to be isolated in culture free from other organisms. He devised liquid and solid culture media which include both serum and blood agar and noted that the organisms grew in clusters called colonies which eventually became visible to the naked eye. He saw that these colonies were characteristic and had defined conditions of growth. After this start the causative organisms of numerous other infectious diseases were isolated and their conditions of growth noted in the same way.

In 1881 Klebs and Loeffler isolated the diphtheria bacillus. The discovery of this organism necessitated a reassessment of the preformed theories of bacterial infection. It was discovered that filtrates of growing cultures of this organism, that is to say material in which the organism had been growing but from which it had been removed by means of filtration, were still able to cause death from diphtheria. This led to the discovery of exotoxins, powerful tissue poisons, often enzymes or ferments, which are

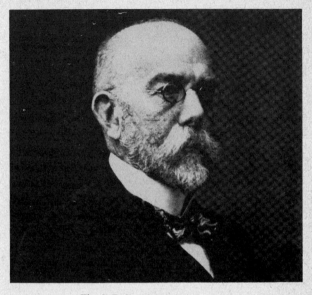

Fig. 3. Robert Koch (1843–1910).

produced by some organisms during growth and which diffuse into the surrounding tissues to be carried through the body in the blood stream, often to produce injurious effects remote from the site of bacterial growth.

In 1890 von Behring showed that diphtheria could be prevented and cured by the administration of serum from a horse convalescent from diphtheria. This was the discovery of antitoxins. In 1891 Ehrlich standardized diphtheria toxin so that its potency could be assessed and the antitoxin measured against it.

At the beginning of this century Ehrlich was investigating the possibility of finding a 'magic bullet', a chemical sufficiently non-toxic to give to a patient but yet capable of destroying all bacteria in his body. In 1910 he discovered an effective chemotherapeutic agent, the arsenical drug

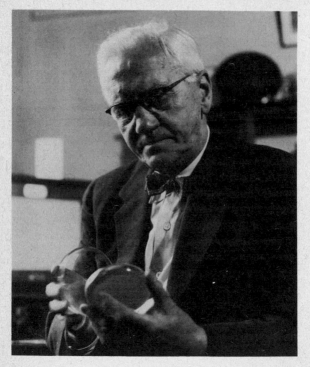

Fig. 4. Sir Alexander Fleming (1881–1955).

salvarsan 606, able to destroy *Treponema pallidum,* and this was used effectively for many years in the treatment of syphilis.

Following Ehrlich's lead the hunt for chemotherapeutic agents was intensified. In 1935 Domagk found the dye prontosil to be effective against streptococci and this drug and many other members of the same chemical family, the sulphonamides, are still widely used to treat suitable infections. In 1929 Fleming discovered penicillin, which after it had been developed in 1940 by Florey and Chain, proved to be a 'magic bullet' that revolutionized the treatment of infections. The outstanding success of penicillin stimulated research that has resulted in the discovery of many chemicals and antibiotics effective against bacteria. At the present time there are a great many antibiotics covering virtually all types of known bacteria.

Virology has developed along broadly similar lines to bacteriology, but necessarily more slowly because of the extremely small size of the infective particles and because they can only multiply within living cells. Pasteur, in 1884, did pioneer work on protection against rabies. Loeffler and Trosch showed filterability of foot-and-mouth disease virus through bacteria-retaining filters in 1898. Culture difficulties have been overcome to a considerable extent by the development of tissue culture techniques, and classification of viruses greatly advanced with the development of the electron microscope.

Some outstanding successes in protection have taken place against virus diseases. Notable amongst these are Jenner's vaccination against smallpox. Theiler's yellow fever vaccine, and the Salk (1953) and Sabin (1955) vaccines for poliomyelitis. More recently vaccines have been used to protect against measles and rubella.

There are sporadic records throughout history of the observation that infection with a particular disease can lead to resistance to reinfection with the same disease. This concept advanced in the eighteenth century following the discovery by Jenner of vaccination against smallpox as mentioned above, and was further developed by Pasteur and many others in the nineteenth century. In the last decade of the nineteenth century it was observed that the serum of immune animals contained factors which neutralized the toxins of the infecting organism. This led rapidly to the development of vaccines against toxin-producing organisms (e.g. diphtheria and tetanus) and to the discovery of the serum components (antibodies) responsible for the neutralization. Meanwhile it became apparent that specific immunity to some diseases such as tuberculosis is mediated not by serum factors, such as antibody, but rather by certain types of cell. We now know that both antibody-mediated and cell-mediated immunity are due to the activity of the lymphoid system, particularly the lymph nodes, spleen and thymus. Modern immunology has revealed that their organs contain numerous distinct subclasses of lymphocyte, some of which are purely regulatory in function, while others are dedicated to the production of antibody, or to one of the ever increasing number of cell-mediated mechanisms. Within the next few years immunologists hope to discover precisely which antibody-mediated or cell-mediated mechanisms are needed to protect against each of the major infectious diseases so that vaccines can be designed to evoke the right kind of response. The development of such 'tailor-made' vaccines will require detailed understanding of how the different mechanisms are regulated. Such knowledge will also facilitate control of rejection of transplanted organs, and of auto-immune disease. It would seem, therefore, that it is in the fields of virology and immunology that major advances will occur in the immediate future.

3 The Structure and Function of Micro-organisms

BACTERIA

Bacteria are minute unicellular organisms ranging in size from 0.3 μm to 14 μm in length (1 μm = 0.001 mm). Ten of the smaller organisms could be placed end to end on the diameter of a red cell, and thirty red cells could fit across the diameter of a pin's head; bacteria cannot therefore be seen with the naked eye and the high-power or oil-immersion lens of a microscope is necessary to make out the shape of individual organisms. Each bacterium, however, is a functioning, living unit, deriving its food from the surroundings in which it finds itself and using this food to manufacture the complex materials necessary for life and reproduction.

Bacteria vary enormously in the substances which they can utilize as food and there are some bacteria nearly everywhere where active steps have not been taken to remove them—in the soil, in hot springs, in the sea, high in the air, in vegetable matter, on animals and in dust—their type depending upon the available foodstuff and the prevailing physical conditions. Some organisms are particular and require exacting conditions in order to flourish, such as the presence of animals or insects upon which they live; when the existence of the organisms depends upon the presence of these animals or insects, they are said to act as vectors or carriers. The organism causing plague is found in rats; fleas bite the rats, become infected with the bacteria, and convey them to human beings. Ridding an area of rats therefore eliminates plague.

Not all bacteria, however, are harmful; indeed many are essential and a great many are useful. A large group of soil bacteria have the power of using atmospheric nitrogen for their growth; as they grow, reproduce and die, organic nitrogenous material is liberated into the soil enriching it and making it available to plants which do not have this power of 'fixing nitrogen'. Bacteria in the soil elaborate vitamins necessary for animal life, and bacteria in the healthy bowel synthesize vitamins essential to human well-being. Bacteria are used to turn curd or cream into cheese, and the products of yet other bacteria turn grape juice into wine and wine into vinegar. These bacterial reactions are carried out commercially and their products are of benefit to mankind.

The term bacteriology therefore covers the study of a vast number of organisms, by far the greater number of which are not met with in medical work and do not cause disease. Those which are encountered in medical bacteriology have, for generations of organisms and centuries of time, become accustomed to living on organic material or animal tisues, and many have lost the power of using simple inorganic substances as a source of food; they have become to a lesser or greater degree parasitic.

Bacteria are of different shapes,* which can be easily

---

*The names of different types of bacteria are derived from Greek and Latin words denoting shape or other characteristic, or, in some cases, from the name of the discoverer of the organism. *Bacterium* is derived from Greek, from the diminutive form of the word *baktron*, a rod. The word, however, has been loosely used for all micro-organisms, whatever their shape. *Coccus* is derived from the Greek word *kokkos,* a berry. *Spirochaete* stems from two Greek words: *speiro,* a coil, and *chaite,* flowing hair. *Bacillus* derives from the Latin *baculus,* a rod. Because of the use of the term bacteria for all organisms, bacillus has been widely used for rod-shaped organisms. Although pathologists have returned to the use of bacterium and prefer it to bacillus, the latter term is still much employed in general medicine.

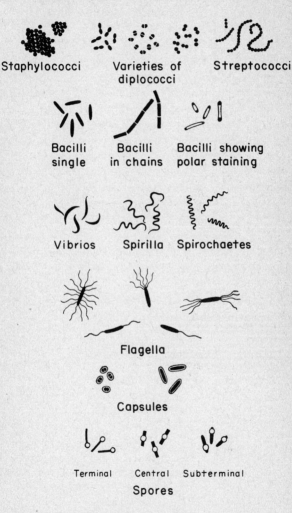

Fig. 5. Some common bacterial shapes and arrangements.

observed when they have been suitably stained and are examined with a high-powered lens on an ordinary microscope. Some varieties are surrounded by a soft jelly-like material, the capsule, which may have a thickness greater than the diameter of the bacteria which it surrounds. Bacteria may be either round, when they are said to be coccoid and are often referred to as *cocci,* or rod-shaped, when they may be called *bacilli.* The term *vibrio* is used to describe a micro-organism which is rigid and has a single curve, e.g. the organism that causes cholera. Longer rigid, curved organisms usually with several spirals are termed *spirilla,* while *spirochaetes* are still longer, but flexible, spiral organisms.

The cocci are divided into several groups in accordance with the way in which they are arranged. They may be arranged in clusters, when they are termed *staphylococci,* or in pairs, when the term *diplococci* is applied to them, or in chains, when they are known as *streptococci.*

The detailed anatomy of bacteria is surprisingly complex for what at first glance appears to be a very simple

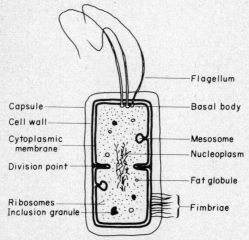

Fig. 6. The anatomy of a bacterium.

structure. Fig. 6 shows diagrammatically the structures that may be demonstrated in common bacteria with the help of an electron microscope. They consist of a rigid cell wall which preserves the shape of the organism, inside which is a thin flexible cytoplasmic membrane which allows diffusion of liquid to take place between the cell cytoplasm and the environment. The cell contents inside the cytoplasmic membrane are liquid, and contain:

1. The nucleoplasm, nuclear material, or deoxyribonucleic acid (DNA), not bounded by a nuclear membrane as occurs with animal and plant cells.
2. Ribosomes, very numerous tiny granules of ribonucleic acid (RNA) or protein.
3. Mesosomes, granules which sometimes may be formed by invagination of the cytoplasmic membrane.
4. Other inclusion granules and fat globules.
5. Division points, partial septa consisting of cell wall and cell membrane which grow completely across the cell at the time of cell division, thus dividing it into two new cells.

Outside the cell wall may be seen in some species one or more of the following:

1. Flagella, hair-like processes which propel species which possess them by a lashing movement.
2. Capsule, a protective gelatinous layer possibly connected with virulence.
3. Fimbriae, short, stout hair-like processes, not concerned with motility, but possibly with adhesion to host cells.

Bacteria require food and water like other living things. Lack of food and absence of water will cause their death. Some bacteria require oxygen and others will flourish only in its absence. Organisms whch require oxygen are termed *aerobes* and those which do not are called *anaerobes*.

Bacteria which need oxygen will be found on the surface of wounds and on skin and mucous membranes, for example the organisms which cause sepsis in wounds or produce colds and other respiratory diseases. Bacteria which do not need oxygen and cannot grow in its presence will particularly affect deep wounds such as stab wounds and deep gunshot wounds; they include the bacteria which cause tetanus and gas gangrene. Sometimes these infections may occur in open wounds because there is a mixed infection, and other bacteria present in the wound use up the oxygen available and so produce conditions in which anaerobic organisms can flourish.

Certain groups of organisms, notably those which cause anthrax and the *Clostridium* group responsible for tetanus and gas gangrene, have, in certain circumstances, the power of developing spores, a highly resistant resting phase which can survive for long periods without food or water and resist wide temperature changes and other adverse environmental conditions which would otherwise be fatal. Like the seeds of plants they can grow and mature again when a suitable temperature, food supply and water become available. Spores may be demonstrated easily by ordinary light microscopy.

VIRUSES

There are three important ways in which viruses differ from other micro-organisms:

1. They are so small that many of them are not visible with a light microscope, though they can be studied with an electron microscope. Viruses vary in size from about 20 to 300 nm whereas staphylococci measure 1000 nm.

2. They possess either DNA or RNA, but never both types of nucleic acid (page 15).

3. Neither viruses nor rickettsiae can grow on lifeless media, but only within living susceptible cells.

Structure

Virus particles consist of a core of nucleic acid (DNA or RNA) surrounded by a protein coat (capsid). Some viruses, e.g. herpesvirus, are enclosed by a further layer or envelope. The capsid protects the nucleic acid and facilitates the attachment of the virus to the host cell, it also contains antigenic material which is specific for each virus type. Electron microscopy studies have demonstrated three types of virus symmetry; cubic, helical and complex. The nucleocapsid of a virus with cubic symmetry is usually icosahedral, i.e. contained by twenty plane faces, e.g. adenovirus. The nucleocapsid of a virus with helical symmetry is elongated and wound in the form of a helix or spiral, e.g. influenza. Those which are neither cubic nor helical are described as having complex symmetry, e.g. smallpox.

RICKETTSIAE AND CHLAMYDIAE
(see pages 185–6)

4 Infection

Infection implies that micro-organisms capable of causing disease have gained access into body tissues, with subsequent establishment and multiplication which actually produces clinical signs of infection. The factors essential to the process of infection are:

1. A pathogenic organism.
2. An entry route into the host.
3. Establishment and multiplication within the host, i.e. the way in which the organism spreads within the body, the type of tissue and conditions in which it can grow and multiply. The susceptibility of the host to infection.
4. An exit route and means of transmission from the host to a new victim.

The organism
A **pathogen** is an organism capable of causing disease. Described as virulent when a very small number produce infection in the host.

A **commensal** is an organism carried harmlessly on or in certain sites but often capable of causing infection when transferred to an abnormal site, e.g. *Escherichia coli,* normally a harmless resident of the gut, causes infection in a wound or the urinary tract.

Routes of entry
Inhalation through the mouth and nose to the respiratory

tract, e.g. the common cold, tuberculosis, diphtheria, influenza, mumps.

Ingestion through the mouth to the alimentary tract, e.g. dysentery, poliomyelitis, salmonellosis, hepatitis A.

Inoculation through the skin or mucous membranes to deeper tissues, e.g. surgery, trauma, insect bites, injections, dressing of surgical wounds. A wider variety of organisms are able to enter the body by this route and to cause conditions ranging from a boil to severe wound infection or virus hepatitis. Healthy intact skin and mucous membranes are natural barriers to infection but when traumatized by accident or surgical procedure, or devitalized by dietary deficiency or an inadequate blood supply, they allow the passage of organisms although they may not appear to be broken.

There are also a few infections which can be transmitted across the placenta, e.g. cytomegalovirus and rubella.

Establishment and reproduction
An organism which has passed a portal of entry stimulates the immune response (page 29) and may be destroyed or may produce an infectious lesion by further progressive invasion of the tissues or by the production of toxins. Tissue invasion may lead to destruction of tissue cells or mechanically important structures, and in some cases infection spreads through the lymphatic channels to the blood stream (the presence of bacteria in the blood stream = bacteraemia and of virus = viraemia; multiplication of bacteria in the blood stream = septicaemia) and once there, may be carried to other organs such as the kidneys or central nervous system to cause further foci of infection. Many micro-organisms produce toxic enzymes which assist in the process of invasion and tissue destruction. Some bacteria, while growing, produce a toxin

(chemical poison) which interferes with some essential process of the host; for example tetanus toxin affects nerve cells in the spinal cord and diphtheria toxin damages both heart muscle and nervous tissue.

To be an effective pathogenic agent an organism must be able to invade a susceptible host; it can do no harm if it cannot get into the tissues no matter how potentially lethal it may be. It must be able to find a suitable place to multiply before it is killed by the defence mechanisms of the body. *Clostridium welchii* is a normal inhabitant of the faeces and soil and frequently gets into wounds. It comparatively rarely causes disease because it can multiply only under anaerobic conditions, that is where there is no free oxygen. In penetrating injuries such as those incurred in war, farming or road traffic accidents, with dirt and dead muscle involved, the conditions become anaerobic, the organisms grow and the disease gas gangrene is produced.

Some organisms, like the haemolytic *Streptococcus,* are relatively unexacting towards the tissues in which they grow, that is to say once they have invaded they can grow and multiply using any tissue in the body as a source of food, and growth will continue unless the organisms are killed by the defences of the body. Others are exacting in their requirements for growth, that is they are more selective and can find the necessary materials only in a particular type of tissue, such as brain tissue in the encephalitis group of viruses or the liver cells in infectious hepatitis. If these exacting organisms do not reach the particular cells in which they can live, they will not produce disease.

Exit and transmission

Having produced the disease in one host, a pathogen, if it is to continue, must be transmitted to another host or the race will die out. This attribute of communicability is a complex one depending upon many factors, of which only a few can be mentioned here.

● The site of the lesion in the infected host, or the place of maximum concentration of the organism, is perhaps the most important factor in communicability of pathogenic organisms. A lesion in the host, as with the haemolytic *Streptococcus* in a case of tonsillitis, can be coughed or

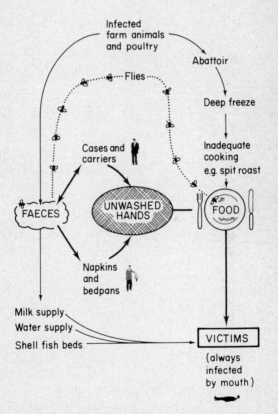

Fig. 7. Transmission of intestinal infections such as *Salmonella* or *Shigella*.

1 AIRBORNE PARTICLES
carry bacteria

2 DIRECT CONTACT via people

STAFF <u>CASES</u>
Stye, Sore throat,
Septic finger,
Boils, D & V

STAFF <u>CARRIERS</u>
from Nose, Throat,
Skin & Intestines

STAFF. <u>POOR TECHNIQUE
AND DISCIPLINE</u>
Long hair and nails
Dirty apron
Touching sterile dressings
Failure to wash hands
Peeking under dressings

<u>PATIENTS</u>
sit on
other beds
share food
etc.

3 PATIENT'S OWN ORGANISMS
Nose / Gut to
wound via fingers

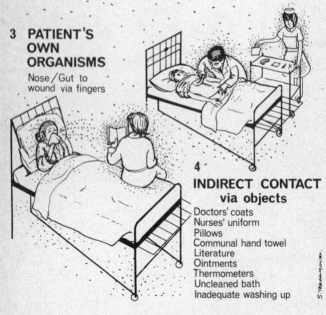

4 INDIRECT CONTACT via objects
Doctors' coats
Nurses' uniform
Pillows
Communal hand towel
Literature
Ointments
Thermometers
Uncleaned bath
Inadequate washing up

Fig. 8. Transmission of pathogenic bacteria in a ward.

breathed into the surrounding air and thus transmitted. Should the same organism be causing mastoid infection there is far less likelihood of it being transmitted because it is bottled up in the bone of the mastoid process.

● The second important factor in the problem of communicability is the length of time an organism capable of causing disease can live outside the human body. Bacteria vary enormously in the length of time that they can survive in unfavourable conditions and their communicability is profoundly affected by this. The organism of tuberculosis can live for many months protected by mucus in sputum even after this has dried, or in the dust away from sunlight, but the gonococcus, the organism causing gonorrhoea, is killed in minutes in dry atmospheric air. Gonorrhoea can therefore be transmitted only by direct contact, from person to person, while tuberculosis can be caught by inhalation of dust from a room which has previously housed a tuberculosis patient.

Routes of transmission of infections
Contact. (a) *Direct contact* from source (see Chapter 11) to victim involving personal contact as in wound dressings, pressure area care, sexually transmitted diseases. Can include endogenous infection (see later) where commensal organisms are carried from a patient's skin to a susceptible site during surgery. (b) *Indirect contact* from source to victim via inanimate objects (fomites) such as contaminated instruments and other equipment or materials such as dressings or clothing.

Airborne. In droplets from one individual to another during coughing or sneezing, e.g. streptococcal infection. In droplet nuclei (bacteria with a protective coat of dried saliva) surviving in dust and thus contaminating surroundings from where they may be inhaled by another individual, e.g. tuberculosis.

Common vehicle. From a communal source to many victims via a contaminated medium such as food or water. *Salmonella* food poisoning is an example of the former, cholera of the latter. Contaminated drug solutions are also in this category as is hepatitis B transmitted via blood products.

Vector-borne via arthropods, i.e. insects and pests such as mosquitoes or Pharoah's ants. This group is of much less importance in the UK than in many other countries.

Contact and airborne routes are most commonly implicated in hospital infection. Understanding of the way in which infection is spread is vital if cross-infection is to be prevented in hospital and community, and the application of this knowledge is discussed in Chapters 11 and 12.

TRANSMISSION OF INFECTION

Endogenous infection is literally 'from within', i.e. the causative organism comes from another part of the victim's own body.

Exogenous infection is infection originating outside the body, i.e. acquired from another person or object, cross infection (see Chapter 11).

Endogenous transfer

A patient or his attendants may inadvertently or carelessly transfer commensal organisms from their normal sites where they are harmless, to another site in the body such as a wound, a pressure sore or tracheostomy, or to equipment such as urine drainage or intravenous infusion apparatus where they can cause infection. For example every patient carries *E. coli* and *Proteus* spp. in the faeces; these easily pass through toilet paper to contaminate the hands; if the hands are not washed the bacteria may be transferred to a vulnerable site to cause infection. During bowel surgery, intestinal organisms may be transferred to the abdominal wall and incision line and cause postoperative wound infection; this is the reason for the meticulous theatre procedure of keeping instruments, swabs and gloves used in contact with the opened bowel separate from those used for the remainder of the operation.

Other commensals are transferred or cause infection only when the surrounding tissue is damaged. For example, *Streptococcus viridans* is always present in the mouth but it can produce dental infection and is forced into the blood stream when a tooth is extracted. If the patient also has diseased heart valves this organism may colonize them and cause subacute bacterial endocarditis.

Symptom-free carriers of pathogenic organisms may disseminate them to other areas where they will cause infection. For example a throat carrier of *Streptococcus pyogenes* (β-haemolytic *Streptococcus* Group A) may develop a septic finger from the same germ if she sucks her grazed or burnt finger to relieve the pain. Many patients, and up to 50% of hospital staff are nasal carriers of *Staphylococcus aureus,* the organism which causes boils and sepsis, although carriage of this organism in some individuals comes and goes in an apparently haphazard way. The system of routinely 'screening' hospital staff for carriage of these two organisms (by taking nose and throat swabs) is generally discontinued. Nasal carriage of staphylococci is acceptable providing individuals realize that contact transmission may be avoided by good hygiene.

From the nose, staphylococci are easily transferred to handkerchiefs, pockets, facecloths, towels, bedding and clothes but particularly to hands, and from any of these contacts to wounds or abrasions can cause infection. Shaving, however skilfully executed, abrades the skin often visibly. If preoperative shaving is scheduled too early, the staphylococci have an opportunity to invade and multiply rapidly in the damaged skin and will be present in very large numbers by the time the patient goes to the operating theatre. The risk of wound infection occurring after incision through such an area is obvious.

Healthy carriers. Patients who have recovered from a disease and who are perfectly well may continue to excrete the pathogenic organism, which causes them no trouble but is a potential source of danger to the community. Such persons are called carriers and are frequently unaware that they are a source of danger and may spread the infectious disease widely, for example a symptom-free nurse or doctor carrying *Streptococcus pyogenes* in the throat; the organisms do not invade but live on the mucous surfaces to be transmitted to another host where conditions may be more suitable for growth and invasion may occur.

It is for this reason that in some occupations involving the handling of food or water, in which pathogenic organisms can be transmitted with ease, the workers are bacteriologically investigated regularly to see if they are carriers of organisms which can be spread in this way, e.g. typhoid excreted in the faeces and spread by unwashed hands.

NORMAL FLORA

The skin and mucous membranes always harbour a variety of micro-organisms because they are in contact with the environment.

Commensal organisms

Commensal organisms are those which normally live in specific sites of the body without invading the tissues or causing infection. Most are not essential to life but they help to maintain the health and normal function of the body; some intestinal commensals, for example, are known to synthesize vitamin K, others to aid in the absorption of nutrients. They are limited in the body to their own commensal sites and in any other site, even any other commensal site, they may act as pathogens or as transient flora. Thus the commensal organisms of the respiratory tract are different from those of the intestinal tract and both are different from those of the skin:

Examples of common commensal organisms

Upper respiratory tract	*Streptococcus viridans*
	Diphtheroids
	Neisseriae catarrhalis
Skin	*Staphylococcus albus*
	Micrococci
	Diphtheroids
Vagina	Lactobacilli
	Coliforms
	Staphylococcus albus
Gut	*Bacteroides* sp.
	Escherichia coli
	Streptococcus faecalis
	Proteus sp.
	Clostridia
	Lactobacilli
	Yeasts

Organisms when constantly found in a particular site are also described as the resident flora, e.g. *Staphylococcus albus* lives in the pores of all healthy, undamaged skin without causing infection; they may be called either skin commensals or resident skin flora.

The transient flora consists of non-pathogenic or potentially pathogenic organisms acquired from the environment. They may inhabit a site from seconds to weeks, but do not ordinarily produce infection or disease and do not become permanently established.

If a commensal organism is transferred to another site in the body it may cause infection, e.g. *Escherichia coli* is a normal inhabitant of the gut where it causes neither disease nor infection; if it is transferred to the bladder it will cause a urinary infection.

In certain conditions the surface normally harbouring mixed flora may become damaged or blocked, allowing organisms usually considered to be of low pathogenicity to invade the damaged mucosa and cause disease, e.g. in bronchitic patients whose respiratory tract mucous membrane has been badly damaged by the disease, normal respiratory tract organisms such as *Haemophilus influenzae* are able to invade and cause acute exacerbations of infection.

It is important that hospital staff are aware of commensal organisms and that both they and their patients carry these organisms which may be transferred from their normal sites in the skin, nose, mouth, throat, respiratory tract, vagina and intestine to another vulnerable site where they may cause infection.

Hospital-acquired (nosocomial) infection. This is infection acquired in hospital, whether originating from a patient, a member of hospital staff or equipment. As mentioned in the introduction, it is responsible for a considerable proportion of infection in hospital patients. It may be either endogenous (self-infection) or exogenous. *Cross-infection* is exogenous transfer from an infected patient to an uninfected one.

Opportunistic infection. All infections are opportunistic but what is generally understood by this term is an infection caused by organisms of low pathogenicity or even commensals which take advantage of lowered immunity however caused, whether by disease, by drugs or by treatment.

5   Immunity

The term immunity in relation to infectious disease derives from the original meaning of the term 'exemption from military service or paying taxes'. It had been recognized from early times that those who had suffered and recovered from infectious disease, e.g. smallpox, measles or diphtheria, were exempt from further attacks of that disease. Such people have developed a *specific immune response* to the infecting organism. The mechanism of this immune response which involves lymphocytes in the lymph nodes and spleen will be discussed in detail later (page 37). Briefly, in the immune individual, re-exposure to the infection results in rapid recognition and destruction of the organisms before they can cause disease. But this is only true for organisms to which the patient has developed an immune response, as a result of either vaccination or previous infection. There is no such thing as generalized immunity to all infectious diseases. Immunity is specific, that is it indicates the ability of the host to resist one particular invader; for example, the fact that we are told that a patient is immune to diphtheria gives us no information as to his immunity to any other unrelated disease, such as measles or tetanus.

The specific immune response is not the only defence against pathogenic organisms. There are a number of *non-specific mechanisms,* not dependent on previous exposure to the organism, which attempt, not always successfully, to prevent the establishment of infection even in non-immune people. It is when these mechanisms fail that the specific immune response becomes of vital importance. These mechanisms will be discussed in the order corresponding roughly to that in which they would act in an individual exposed to infection for the first time.

Non-specific defence mechanisms
   1. Prevention of invasion:
     a. Skin.
     b. Mucous surfaces.
     c. Secretions.
     d. Mechanical arrangement of structures.
   2. Non-specific mechanisms following invasion:
     Inflammation and phagocytosis.
   3. The Complement System.

Specific immune responses
   1. Induction of the immune response.
   2. Mechanisms of action of the specific immune response:
     a. B-lymphocytes and antibody production.
     b. T-lymphocytes and cell-mediated immunity.

NON-SPECIFIC DEFENCE MECHANISMS

Prevention of invasion
The body is surrounded by organisms, both pathogenic and non-pathogenic, since they are present on everything we touch and eat and the air we breathe; therefore the skin and mucous surfaces must form the first line of defence.

The skin. The skin has often been said to be impermeable to invasion by pathogenic organisms, but this is only a half-truth. The skin, unlike a sheet of Cellophane, is a complex structure constantly renewing itself and containing hair follicles, sweat and sebaceous glands. The hair follicles and sweat glands harbour many organisms

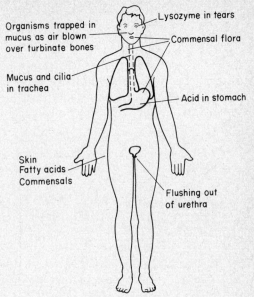

Fig. 9. Non-specific barriers to infection.

which it is impossible to remove in spite of the most meticulous treatment, and pathogenic organisms frequently invade from these sites. Axillary abscesses and beard infections are common results of such infection and are difficult to treat. Intact skin does, however, form a barrier against many pathogenic bacteria, and its secretions have antibacterial properties.

Mucous surfaces. In certain situations where the number of bacteria is high the surfaces are moistened with a mucous secretion to entrap the organisms until they can be removed; the nose, mouth and vagina are good examples of this.

Secretions. All organs in the body which are in contact with the external environment produce secretions. These are most appreciable in places where there is potentially the greatest danger of bacterial invasion. These secretions act in two ways:

1. *By mechanical action.* Secretions of the bronchi entrap organisms and the flow of secretion is moved away from the alveoli by the action of the cilia on the bronchial walls. Tears also wash organisms away from the conjunctivae.

2. *By chemical action of their constituents.* These secretions may be acid, like sweat, adult vaginal secretion and gastric juice, or contain fatty acids, like sweat, or be strongly alkaline, like bile. Abrupt changes from an acid to an alkaline environment are known, for example, to keep the bacterial flora of the alimentary canal in check. Tears and certain other mucosal secretions, for example nasal mucus and saliva, contain an active antibacterial substance, lysozyme. When cells are infected by viruses they may release *interferon,* which increases the resistance of neighbouring cells to the infection.

The mechanical arrangement of structures. As air is inspired it is taken in at high velocity as if by a vacuum cleaner, and this air may contain many pathogenic organisms. The arrangement of the mucus-covered turbinate bones in the nose is such that the air impinges upon them and bacteria stick to the mucous surfaces. The speed of flow of air is considerably reduced, due to the increasing area of the bronchial passages, with the result that by the time the air reaches the alveoli it is travelling very slowly and contains very few organisms. The mucus, swept by the cilia up the air passages into the pharynx, is subsequently swallowed and many of the organisms are killed by the acid in the gastric juice.

The direction of the bronchi may have something to do with the localization of lung infections and the short straight auditory tubes in infants may play a part in the greater frequency of middle ear infections in comparison with infections in adults. The shortness of the urethra in the female compared with that of the male accounts for the ease with which organisms can ascend to the bladder and cause cystitis.

Non-specific defence mechanisms following invasion

If an organism succeeds in getting through the non-specific barriers above, and so enters the tissues, further non-specific defence mechanisms are activated. These are still not dependent on the specific immune response but, as will be seen later, their efficiency is greatly enhanced by it.

Non-specific inflammation and phagocytosis. Most organisms, once they have entered the tissues, will cause inflammation. The signs of inflammation are heat, redness, swelling and tenderness or pain. These signs are similar whether the tissue irritant is a *Staphylococcus,* a sterile splinter or a chemical irritant.

Capillary dilatation results in an outpouring of fluid, white cells and some red cells from the blood vessels into the tissues. This outpouring of cells and serum is important, since it brings them into contact with the organisms. Serum contains substances which attach non-specifically to the surfaces of many organisms. This can lead, after further interactions with yet another series of serum factors called the *complement system,* to engulfment of the organisms by phagocytic cells (macrophages and polymorphonuclear leucocytes).

The complement system (abbreviated as C′)

The complement system is in many ways analogous to the clotting system. Thus both systems consist of numerous enzymes and co-factors which interact with each other in an orderly sequence, often called an 'enzyme cascade'. When the clotting system is activated the result of this complex series of reactions is a clot. When the complement system is activated, there are several important consequences which help in the destruction of infecting organisms. These mechanisms will be described later. First we must consider how the complement system is activated.

Activation of the complement system. Just as the clotting system can be activated by contact with glass, so the complement system can be activated by contact with the surfaces of some organisms (see Fig. 10). This type of complement activation is called the 'alternative pathway'. The other type of complement activation, called the 'classical pathway' because it was the first to be described, involves antibody and will be considered later with the 'specific' immune response. The two pathways lead, via 'enzyme cascades', to the activation of the most important complement component, known as C_3.

The antimicrobial effects of the complement system (see Figs 10 and 11). Complement components from the blood will leak out into a site of inflammation and infection. Once activated at such a site the following things may happen:

1. The organisms may become coated with derivatives of one of the complement components known as C_3. This causes the organisms to adhere strongly to the membranes of phagocytic cells which have a binding site or 'receptor' for C_3. This attachment of the organisms to phagocytes greatly increases the efficiency with which they are engulfed. Indeed C_3 is so important that congenital absence of it leads to rapid death from infection.

2. Other components are then modified enzymically and become active as chemotaxins. That is to say that they attract more phagocytic cells to the site of infection.

3. Another group of complement components can lyse cell membranes *(The Lytic pathway)*. These are the factors which lyse red blood cells when an unmatched blood

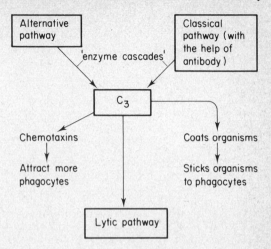

Fig. 10. Activation of the complement system.

transfusion has been given. A few species of bacteria and viruses can be killed by this lytic pathway, but this function of complement, although the most well-known, is not as important as the binding to membranes via C_3 and congenital absence of one of the factors involved can be symptomless.

The destruction of engulfed organisms. Once engulfed by phagocytes (polymorphs or macrophages) with the help of the alternative complement pathway and C_3, the organisms are contained within membrane-bound vacuoles called phagosomes, where they are exposed to a variety of microbicidal mechanisms. Then the contents of the lysosomes are emptied into the phagosomes. Lysosomes contain a number of digestive enzymes which help to eliminate the organisms. Occasionally the situation is reversed and the organisms kill the phagocytes. Pus is an accumulation of living and dead phagocytes, other blood and tissue cells, cell debris and bacteria.

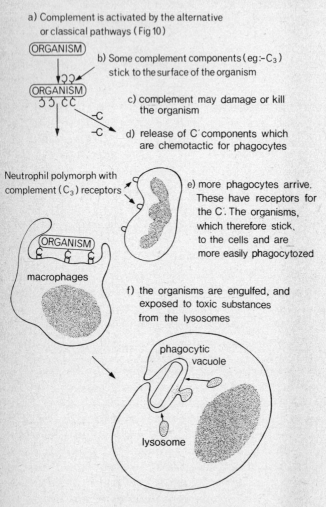

a) Complement is activated by the alternative or classical pathways (Fig 10)

ORGANISM

b) Some complement components (eg:-C_3) stick to the surface of the organism

ORGANISM

c) complement may damage or kill the organism

d) release of C′ components which are chemotactic for phagocytes

Neutrophil polymorph with complement (C_3) receptors

e) more phagocytes arrive. These have receptors for the C′. The organisms, which therefore stick, to the cells and are more easily phagocytozed

ORGANISM

macrophages

f) the organisms are engulfed, and exposed to toxic substances from the lysosomes

phagocytic vacuole

lysosome

Fig. 11. Phagocytosis.

THE SPECIFIC IMMUNE RESPONSE

While the struggle outlined above is going on, the lymphocytes in the lymphoid system are beginning to mount the specific immune response, which then comes to the aid of the non-specific mechanisms.

The induction of the immune response (See Fig. 12)
Stage 1. Every organism is made up of a unique mixture of cell wall components, cytoplasm, enzymes and perhaps toxins. Most of these molecules are unlike anything present in the patient's own tissues and so are recognized as 'foreign'. These are known as *antigens*. Antigens from the infecting organism pass along the lymphatics, free or in macrophages, to the draining lymph nodes.

Stage 2. In the draining lymph node, the antigens come into contact with the surfaces of lymphocytes. Each lymphocyte carries on its surface *receptors* which enable it to recognize one particular type of antigen. When antigen attaches to lymphocytes with receptors of the right specificity the cells begin to proliferate. This proliferation leads to a great increase in the number of lymphocytes able to recognize the antigen in question.

Stage 3. The lymphocytes leave the lymph node via the efferent lymphatics and travel to the site of the infection via the blood stream. Here they assist in the struggle against the infection in a number of ways which are described in the next section.

Mechanisms of action of the specific immune response
B-lymphocytes and antibody production. The lymphocytes discussed above are of two kinds, B-lymphocytes (B-cells) and T-lymphocytes (T-cells).

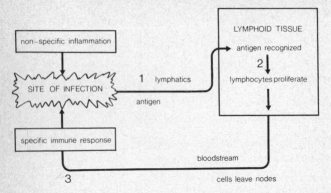

Fig. 12. Induction of the immune response. Numbers refer to the stages of induction.

The B-lymphocytes are the precursors of *antibody-producing cells* (plasma cells). Plasma cells release molecules similar to the antigen-recognizing receptors already described and these molecules, which are referred to as *antibody,* accumulate in the serum and may be present in astonishingly large quantities. Antibodies are subdivided into several classes, each of which has different properties; they are referred to collectively as immunoglobulins. Each antibody molecule has the ability to combine specifically with more antigen of the kind which induced the proliferative lymphocyte response in the draining lymph node. In fact since each antibody molecule may have several antigen-specific combining sites, it may be able to attach to several antigen molecules.

The major types (classes) of antibody
IgG. The most abundant class of antibody in the serum is immunoglobulin G (IgG). Each molecule of IgG has two antigen-binding sites. IgG crosses the placenta and so is present in babies at birth.

IgM. The other major class in serum is IgM. It is larger than IgG and each molecule has ten antigen-binding sites.

Two other classes of antibody are only present in small quantities in serum and have rather special properties:

IgA is actively secreted into the gut, bronchi, tears and saliva. It may help to block adherence of organisms and uptake of antigens from the food.

IgE is the immunoglobulin class responsible for hay fever, because, rather than circulating in the blood, it attaches itself to mast cells and basophils, which are triggered to release compounds such as histamine in the presence of the antigen to which the IgE binds.

Fig. 13 illustrates the ways in which antibody (mainly IgM and IgG) protect the host.

1. By combining with the active parts of toxins, such as those released in diphtheria or tetanus, antibody can neutralize their effects.

2. Viruses have to attach to cells before they can enter them and cause infection. Antibody can cover the virus and block its ability to do this, e.g. influenza virus.

3. Since each antibody molecule can combine with more than one antigen molecule, antibody can agglutinate antigens or antigen-carrying organisms. Such big clumps of, for instance, small viruses are more easily engulfed by phagocytic cells.

4. Some organisms become coated with complement (page 33) by means of a direct interaction with various serum factors. Other organisms do not activate complement until antibody molecules have attached to their surfaces. After this has occurred, the antigen-bound antibody itself can activate the complement system (Classical pathway, see Fig. 10), which leads to attachment of complement to the surface of the organism. Some organisms are lysed by these complement components (Lytic pathway, see Fig. 10).

5. Receptors for complement (C_3 receptors) are found on the membranes of phagocytic cells (page 33). There are also receptors for the free end of antibody molecules (F_C receptors) and the 'opsonized' organism thus sticks firmly to macrophages and polymorphs which can then phagocytose the organism very efficiently.

6. Antibody (IgA) is secreted into the bronchi, the gut and tears and so can reinforce the non-specific barriers such as mucus and cilia (page 30). Antibody is also secreted in the maternal milk and some subclasses (IgG) can cross the placenta so that babies are protected for the first few months of life by the mother's antibody. Meanwhile they begin to develop their own immune responses.

T-lymphocytes and cell-mediated immunity
The T-lymphocytes are so called because they are dependent, particularly in early life, on the presence of the thymus gland. These lymphocytes are absent in the rare children with congenital absence of the thymus and such children have very low resistance to infection, due primarily to loss of *cell-mediated immunity*. As the name suggests, cell-mediated immunity involves the direct interaction of T-lymphocytes with antigen. Unlike the B-cell, where antibody is the antigen-recognizing receptor and the mechanism is known, the T-cell receptor and the way in which it recognizes antigen is not yet fully understood.

Two important ways in which T-cell mediated immunity protects the host are illustrated in Fig. 14.

1. When a T-cell encounters the antigen which its receptors recognize, it may release mediators known collectively as lymphokines. The lymphokines make macrophages in the vicinity become activated. This involves a number of complex metabolic changes, the most

Mechanisms of the specific immune response

B – lymphocytes

antigen

antigen recognition

proliferation
and maturation

antibody secretion

plasma cells

Effects of antibody

1. neutralization of toxins

2. neutralization of virus

3. agglutination

4. killing of organisms:
   activation of complement
   system

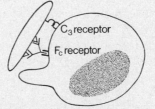

5. opsonization
   (enhancement of
   phagocytosis)

C₃ receptor

F_c receptor

6. antibody may be present in mucous membrane secretions

Fig. 13. B-lymphocyte mechanisms in the specific immune response.
Numbers refer to those on pages 39–40.

Mechanisms of the specific immune response

T – lymphocytes

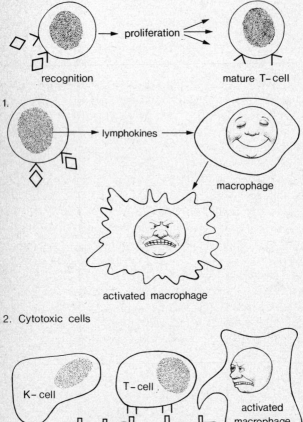

2. Cytotoxic cells

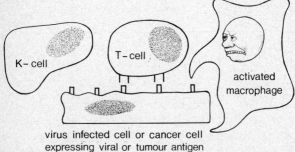

Fig. 14. T-lymphocyte mechanisms in the specific immune response. Numbers refer to those on pages 42–3.

important of which is an increased ability to destroy micro-organisms. For example tubercle bacilli, even when coated with antibody and complement, appear not to be killed by normal macrophages but activated macrophages can destroy them. This is also the mechanism of defence against leprosy.

2. T-cells and their 'assistants', the activated macrophages, are also able to recognize and damage cells which have become foreign to the host. For instance, virus-infected cells may express viral antigens on to their surface. The cell-mediated response can recognize these antigens and help to localize the infection by attacking such cells and interrupting the virus replication cycle. This mechanism is of particular importance for defence against viruses such as varicella–zoster which can pass directly from cell to cell without being released into the body fluids where they would be exposed to antibody. This is why it is common to see an exacerbation of varicella–zoster when T-cell function is compromised, e.g. in patients undergoing cytotoxic therapy.

Similarly, cells which are undergoing mutations or becoming cancerous may alter antigenically and evoke a cell-mediated response. Another recently described cell type which is neither a T-cell nor a B-cell may also be involved in this type of reaction. It is known as a killer or K-cell and can destroy cells which are already coated with antibody.

SKIN TESTS

If a quantity of antigen too small to cause non-specific inflammation is introduced into the skin of a non-immune individual nothing can be seen at the site of injection.

If the individual has developed a cell-mediated immune response to the antigen in question, T-lymphocytes and macrophages accumulate at the site of injection and cause inflammation, swelling and induration, reaching a peak at 48 or 72 h. This phenomenon, referred to as delayed hypersensitivity is the basis of the tuberculin test. It can be used to test for cell-mediated responsiveness to many other antigens apart from tuberculin

However, at least two other phenomena can occur at such a skin-test site, and these must be distinguished from delayed hypersensitivity.

Thus if the individual has IgE antibody to the test antigen (see page 39) there may be an immediate reaction within minutes due to mediator release from mast cells. Similarly, if there is much IgG or IgM, antigen/antibody complexes may form in the blood vessel walls at the test site. This causes inflammation within 8 h. which then declines. Thus tuberculin tests should always be read at 72 h.

SUMMARY OF THE IMMUNE RESPONSE

The last few pages have described the most important mechanisms which contribute to the immune response. It is essential to realize that during an actual infection all of these mechanisms will play some part, so that an analysis of what is happening at any one time becomes very complicated. This is partly because they are all inter-related. For instance macrophages are important for both antibody responses and cell-mediated responses, and the presence of some antibody and complement is probably essential for the optimal functioning of cell-mediated responses.

If the various mechanisms are understood it is possible to predict the sequence of events in a particular disease. For example, a virus enters by the mouth or respiratory tract and initially infects the mucosa in one of these sites. Physical barriers oppose this, and secreted antibody may prevent it in the immune individual. If the virus succeeds in establishing itself in the cells of the mucosa, it replicates and is released into the blood stream. This is a critical stage. If antibody is present the virus is neutralized, agglutinated and coated with antibody and complement so that it adheres to phagocytes in the blood, liver and spleen via the complement and antibody receptors. It is then rapidly removed and destroyed. In the absence of antibody, the tiny virus particles are not efficiently removed and survive to reach their target organ (the nervous system in poliomyelitis etc.). They then enter cells again, so that antibody is of little help except to mop up any further released virus; the cell-mediated response must take over by recognizing infected cells and limiting local spread. Thus all the mechanisms discussed have occurred in one disease.

NEW DEVELOPMENTS

Immunology is a very rapidly developing field and there are a number of advances of which the reader should be aware, in addition to the very simplified scheme described earlier in this chapter.

Lymphocyte sub-populations
The simple division of lymphocytes into B-cells and T-cells is no longer sufficient. There are several different types of T-cell and these differ in function. Some mediate the various types of response, whereas others regulate or suppress them. Some types of T-cell are involved in regulation of antibody production by B-cells.

Macrophage sub-populations
Macrophages are very heterogeneous. Functional sub-populations are beginning to be defined, with differing microbicidal or tumoricidal activity.

Interferon
Interferon is mentioned on page 166 as an antiviral agent,

released by infected cells. It is now clear that there are many related types of interferon which play a complex regulatory role in cellular processes, which need not involve viruses. There has been some excitement about possible anti-tumour effects.

Transfer factor

If normal leucocytes are lysed and dialysed, the dialysate contains a factor which appears to be able to correct defects in cell-mediated immunity in some children with congenitally abnormal responses, and in certain disseminated infections. Its mode of action is mysterious, but trials are in progress in leprosy and leishmaniasis.

Immunogenetics

When studying the antigens against which the immune response is directed during graft rejection, it was noticed that most of these were coded for only one chromosome, in a closely linked group of loci now known as the major histocompatibility complex (MHC). This stretch of DNA codes for several immunologically relevant molecules and in particular for two major classes of cell surface glycopeptide. Apart from their role in graft rejection these glycopeptides are involved in 'communication' between lymphoid cells, and between macrophages and lymphocytes. Moreover, antigens are recognized in association with these glycopeptides on the surfaces of antigen-presenting or infected cells. Thus they may have fundamental regulatory roles in deciding *which antigens* should evoke responses and which *type of response* should be activated.

There are many different alleles which can occur at each locus within the major histocompatibility complex. These code for subtly different variants of these important glycopeptides. Thus in some ways it resembles the blood group system, although far more complex. Possession of some of these variants is associated with an increased incidence of certain diseases. Since the human major histocompatibility complex has been named the 'HLA' system, such diseases are described as HLA-linked. Ankylosing spondylitis is the most clear-cut example.

Monoclonal antibodies

It is now possible to fuse antibody-producing cells with tumour cells, to make an 'immortal' clone of dividing antibody secreting cells, known as a hybridoma. In theory such a hybridoma could go on making antibody of one specificity forever, providing unlimited quantities of a perfectly standardized reagent. Such monoclonal reagents are more specific than conventional antibodies, such as are derived from a single antibody secreting cell. Conventional antibodies are mixtures derived from large numbers of B-cells of slightly different specificity.

These monoclonal antibodies are revolutionizing biology because they provide astonishingly precise probes for analysing the structure of complex organic molecules. Moreover their clinical importance is becoming apparent, because selected monoclonals can be used to identify leukaemia cells in blood samples, or the origin of tumour cells in sections, and they will gradually begin to be used for diagnostic procedures in microbiology laboratories, or for assay of drugs, hormones and serum constituents.

VACCINATION AND IMMUNIZATION

Any infectious disease may cause serious complications, even death, and all have some effect on the community in which they occur, for instance school closure or quarantine restrictions or loss of working time. One measure taken to prevent outbreaks and to protect populations against certain diseases is immunization.

Immunization, that is, artificially induced immunity, may be short-term passive immunity or active immunity when the production of specific antibody is stimulated in response to administration of specific antigen but without causing a clinical attack of the disease.

Passive immunity

Serum from a convalescent person or animal contains specific antibody. This is given:

1. *Therapeutically* to a patient who has already succumbed to the same disease and is not producing sufficient antibody to combat the causative organism or its toxins, e.g. diphtheria antitoxin, antitetanus serum.

2. *Protectively* to a person already at high risk from infection. For instance, susceptible children with conditions such as leukaemia or congenital heart abnormalities are given immunoglobulin (antibody) from a convalescent case, if another child in the ward develops measles. They would be most likely to catch measles, with very serious consequences, if not protected in this way. Similarly, specific hepatitis B immunoglobulin may be given to a member of staff accidentally inoculated with blood from a patient with hepatitis B.

Such immunity is instant but short-term.

Active immunity

Active immunity is induced by:

1. Suffering from the disease.
2. Inoculation of the organism, or the product of the organism (toxin), responsible for the disease. The organism has to be treated so that it induces the immune response but does not produce the disease.

Vaccines and antitoxins are produced by:

1. Killing the organism, e.g. typhoid.

2. Attenuation of the organism, e.g. BCG, poliomyelitis. Attenuated strains have lost the power to produce invasive infection but induce the same antibody response as fully virulent strains.

3. Modification of exotoxins, e.g. diphtheria, tetanus. In diseases purely due to toxaemia the only antigen capable of inducing the immune response is the exotoxin so that in these diseases it is not necessary to inoculate the complete organism. The exotoxin causes the disease and therefore has to be modified before administration. This is usually done by treatment with formaldehyde and the modified toxin is called *toxoid*. Toxoid induces the same immune response as toxin but does not result in symptoms of the disease.

Length of protection
An attack of a disease or immunization against it does not necessarily confer life-long immunity. The length of protection time varies, but antibody level and therefore resistance to attack is always greatest immediately after recovery from the acute phase of the disease. In streptococcal infections the antibody level fails relatively quickly and further attacks are not uncommon. In other diseases such as measles the antibody level declines equally rapidly but the immune response remains and it is unusual to have more than one attack of the disease. Some infections such as the common cold appear to recur but this is due to the multiplicity of strains of the virus, each antigenically different but each producing comparable symptoms. That is, a series of different colds is due to different antigenic strains not to repeated attacks of the same illness.

Immunization schedules
The diseases against which routine immunization is advised by the Department of Health and Social Security (United Kingdom) are diphtheria, pertussis, tetanus, poliomyelitis,

measles and tuberculosis. Rubella (German measles) immunization should be offered to all girls at the age of 12–13 years who have not had the natural disease because, if they suffer the disease during pregnancy, there is a risk of the infection producing congenital malformations in their babies.

It is unwise to attempt to immunize babies under six months of age because:

1. The immune-response-producing mechanism is not fully developed at this age and therefore antibody production is poor.

2. A high level of maternally transmitted antibody (transplacental and in the milk) may also adversely affect the baby's ability to form antibodies.

3. Severe reactions to the immunizing agents are more likely to occur before this age. On the other hand, it is advisable to immunize children as early as possible because protection is needed most between the ages of one and four years as judged by infectious diseases notification figures.

To reduce the number of visits and the number of injections to a minimum, combined vaccines consisting of mixtures of compatible immunizing agents should be used whenever possible. Fig. 15 provides an acceptable schedule.

Vaccination against smallpox is no longer recommended as a routine procedure in early childhood and is only recommended for staff working in designated smallpox units.

Routine vaccination against rabies is not usually considered necessary because the long incubation period allows time for prophylactic active immunization after exposure to an infected animal or to the disease.

In order to avoid the risk of travellers introducing infectious diseases, many countries insist upon travellers holding valid immunization certificates on entry. Countries

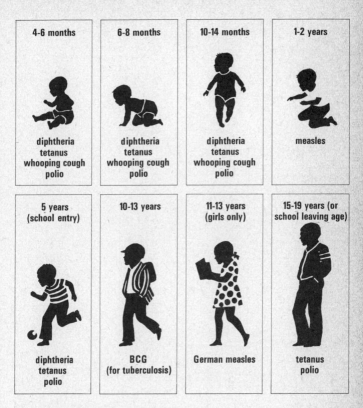

Fig. 15. The immunization schedule recommended in Great Britain. (By kind permission of *Which?*).

vary a good deal in their requirements, but many require evidence of immunization against cholera and yellow fever. Where these are required immunizations are valid internationally for six months for cholera and ten years for yellow fever.

Detailed information on recommendations and requirements for immunization is given in the following publications:

Department of Health and Social Security (1972) *Immunization against Infectious Diseases*. London: HMSO.

World Health Organization. *Vaccination Requirements for International Travel*. Geneva.

6 Chemotherapy

Treatment of infectious disease by destroying invading micro-organisms within the body was unknown before the pioneer work of Ehrlich at the beginning of this century. In 1904 he succeeded in curing experimental trypanosomiasis (sleeping sickness) by using a dye, trypan red, and in 1910 he showed that the organic arsenical compound salvarsan 606 could cure certain protozoal and spirochaetal infections in man. This latter substance was used successfully in the treatment of syphilis for many years. This was virtually the extent of specific drug therapy against infection for the following 25 years.

The modern era may be said to have begun in 1935 when Domagk reported some successes against bacterial diseases due to the β-haemolytic *Streptococcus* with prontosil, a drug of the sulphonamide group. Since 1935 various other drugs belonging to this family have been synthesized to give a wider range of activity against more bacteria, greater potency, less toxicity, and different physicochemical properties, but the action of the whole group is fundamentally the same, depending on the sulphanilamide content. The action of these drugs is bacteriostatic, rather than bactericidal; the organisms are prevented from growing and multiplying and the normal defence mechanisms of the body are enabled to deal with the infection.

In 1940 Woods and Fildes formulated an hypothesis that bacteriostasis occurs by blocking metabolic pathways of the organism. This was based on Woods' observation on the mode of action of sulphonamide. We have seen that bacteria vary enormously in the nutritive material which they can use for building up into bacterial protoplasm and enzymes for breaking down to provide the energy necessary for this synthesis. Some organisms provided with atmospheric nitrogen and carbon can synthesize complex bacterial proteins by an enormous number of chemical changes, each change being catalysed or brought about by a specific enzyme, the process forming a chain of reactions culminating in new bacterial bodies. Loss of an enzyme along this chain of reactions will cause a break in the chain and growth will stop unless the substance is provided in the form of another material, chemically 'nearer' in the chain of the reactions to the bacterial protoplasm, in which case the need for the missing enzyme is eliminated. A substance or chemical group which is necessary for growth of a particular organism is known as an essential metabolite for that organism.

All bacteria which are sensitive to the sulphonamides, and that is a wide range of organisms, require as an essential metabolite *para*-aminobenzoic acid which is a precursor of folic acid. This substance is very similar to sulphanilamide, but sulphanilamide is not biologically active and it cannot take the place of an essential metabolite in the chain of reactions. It is, however, sufficiently similar to react with the enzyme of the bacterial body which uses *para*-aminobenzoic acid. Once the enzyme has reacted with the drug the chain of reactions becomes blocked and growth cannot take place.

In order to produce an effective concentration in the blood, a high dose is given initially, and subsequently reduced to a maintenance level which ensures a high ratio of sulphonamide to *para*-aminobenzoic acid.

If the organism is to survive in a medium flooded with sulphanilamide it must either make its own *para*-aminobenzoic acid from simpler substances or adopt a chain of reactions bypassing the reaction needing *para*-aminobenzoic acid. Both these courses are possible if the bacteria are given sufficient time; they can be trained to do without the essential metabolite and once this resistant strain has been produced, further sulphonamide treatment is useless. It is essential therefore to prevent pathogenic organisms from making these metabolic adjustments, and this is done by flooding the tissues with a sulphonamide. Inadequate therapy and small doses are dangerous, because once a resistant strain has been produced, there is evidence that even in a different host it remains resistant.

A more recent drug, *trimethoprim,* has been shown to potentiate the action of sulphonamides by blocking the metabolism of folic acid to folinic acid—the next step to that blocked by sulphonamide. Combinations of these drugs (e.g. cotrimoxazole) are synergistic, that is, they are more effective against sensitive infections than either drug alone or than the simple sum of their separate activities would suggest. Trimethoprim is usually prescribed in combination since by itself the drug has low activity and bacteria rapidly develop resistance to it. However, it is used alone for some urinary tract infections.

Para-aminosalicylic acid (PAS) stands in the same relationship to salicylic acid as the sulphonamides do to *para*-aminobenzoic acid. The growth of virulent tubercle bacilli is stimulated by salicylic acid and inhibited by the closely related substance *para*-aminosalicylic acid.

ANTIBIOTICS

Antibacterial substances which are produced by living cells are known as antibiotics. It has been known for many years that substances produced by various groups of bacteria or moulds will inhibit the growth of other groups of organisms. Many of these substances are also toxic to animal tissues but a few are sufficiently selective in their action against micro-organisms to be used as therapeutic agents. It was not until 1929 that the full importance of these substances began to be recognized.

Penicillin

In 1928, Fleming noticed that colonies of staphylococci were 'dissolved' round a mould of *Penicillin notatum* which was growing by accident on a culture plate. From this mould Florey later extracted the active substance penicillin, the pure form of which is now known as benzyl-penicillin. It is supplied as the sodium or potassium salt and is also known as soluble or crystalline penicillin.

Penicillin is very selective in its action and in general it may be said that the Gram-positive cocci and bacilli, the pathogenic Gram-negative cocci and the spirochaetes are sensitive, while the Gram-negative rods and the viruses are penicillin resistant.

Those organisms which are resistant to penicillin are resistant either because they can grow unharmed in penicillin or because they themselves produce a substance, penicillinase, which destroys penicillin. It is for this reason that treatment by penicillin of a mixed infection due to a sensitive and a resistant organism so often fails. One sees it frequently in varicose ulcers or external ear infections. The primary organism is sensitive, but the lesion becomes secondarily infected with a penicillin-destroying organism.

In all sensitive cultures there are a few organisms which are relatively more resistant than the rest; these arise naturally. In the presence of concentrations of penicillin sufficient to kill the majority, this minority are not killed and they multiply; in this way a resistant strain is established. Since the regular use of penicillin the number of resistant strains of some organisms, particularly staphylococci, has enormously increased; this is why chemotherapy should be reserved for serious infections.

Penicillin has very low toxicity so that very large doses can be given. It is, however, easily inactivated, the newer,

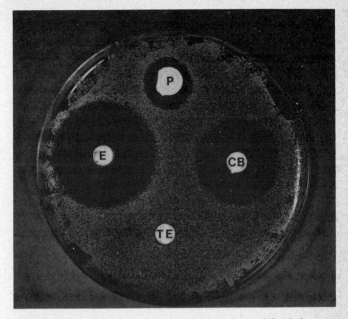

Fig. 16. Estimation of antibiotic sensitivity. Culture of *Staphylococcus aureus*. Sensitivity indicated by inhibition of growth around discs. P = penicillin; CB = methicillin; TE = tetracycline; and E = erythromycin.

purer preparations less so than the older ones. The drug is unstable in solution and its activity rapidly diminishes. Such things as heat, acids, alkalis, alcohol, metals, oxidizing agents, disinfectants and time readily destroy its potency. The dry salt of benzylpenicillin is, however, stable at room temperature. Because of its inactivation by acids, benzylpenicillin is partially destroyed in the stomach, but it may successfully be given by mouth if in sufficiently large doses. For severe infections, however, it must be given by intramuscular injection. It is now considered bad therapy to prescribe small doses of penicillin for local application, e.g. in toothpaste, chewing gum or lozenges which may encourage resistant strains of bacteria and make the patient allergic to the drug.

Penicillin diffuses rapidly through the tissues and an adequate blood level is reached within 15 minutes of an intramuscular injection; the excretion rate through the kidneys is also rapid so that however large a dose of crystalline penicillin is given the level falls quickly, and after three hours another dose must be given if an adequate level is to be maintained.

Three-hourly injections were wearisome to the patient in hospital and extremely difficult in domiciliary cases. Then preparations were developed which are stable in the presence of acid (i.e. phenoxymethylpenicillin or penicillin V) and can thus survive passage through the stomach when given by mouth. These are absorbed from the small gut in an active form; however, none of these is quite as effective as benzylpenicillin, which should always be given for severe sensitive infections.

The basic nucleus of penicillin, 6-aminopenicillanic acid, has been isolated (Batchelor *et al.* 1959) and it is now possible to produce semi-synthetic modifications. These modifications include:

1. Acid-stable compounds which can be taken by mouth: flucloxacillin, ampicillin, carfecillin.
2. Penicillinase-resistant compounds which will be active in penicillinase-producing staphylococcal infections: methicillin, flucloxacillin.
3. Compounds with broad spectrum activity: ampicillin, amoxycillin.
4. Compounds active against *Pseudomonas aeruginosa*: carbenicillin, azlocillin, mezlocillin, ticarcillin, piperacillin.

Carbenicillin was the first penicillin compound to become available that had a useable degree of activity against *Pseudomonas aeruginosa*. However, its activity was low and large daily doses of 20–30 g, which had to be given intravenously, were necessary. Recent developments in penicillin research have been aimed at the production of compounds with greater anti-pseudomonas activity. New drugs that have the same general antibacterial spectrum as carbenicillin, but greater weight for weight activity are azlocillin, mezlocillin, ticarcillin and piperacillin. Carfecillin is a variety of penicillin, which is acid stable and on absorption from the gut is changed to carbenicillin. It is excreted in the urine and, because of the concentrating action of the kidney, an effective amount to treat *Pseudomonas* infection of the urinary tract is attained. It is not effective to treat infection at other sites in the body.

The penicillins all act by interfering with bacterial cell wall synthesis.

The cephalosporins

The cephalosporins are a family of antibiotics broadly similar chemically and in their spectrum of activity to penicillin. Like penicillin a part of the molecule can be substituted in various ways to produce compounds with differing antibacterial action. Recently a number of derivatives with increased effectiveness against Gram-negative organisms have been produced, cefamandole, cefoxitin and cefuroxime are examples of these. An important indication for the use of these drugs is hyper-sensitivity to penicillin, but care must be exercised as such patients are often sensitive to the cephalosporins as well.

Aminoglycosides

Since the discovery of penicillin there have been numerous other antibacterial substances produced from soil bacteria, notably the *Streptomyces* group, of which streptomycin was one of the first.

Streptomycin inhibits the growth of nearly all pathogenic organisms with the exception of the spore-bearing organisms, fungi, viruses and rickettsiae; it has therefore the advantage over benzylpenicillin of inhibiting the Gram-negative rods including the coli-typhoid-dysentery group, and also *Mycobacterium tuberculosis*.

Streptomycin is given by intramuscular injection because, although it is more stable than penicillin, it is not absorbed through the gut. Its excretion by the kidneys is not so rapid as penicillin and adequate blood levels can be maintained for 6 to 12 h. after a single injection.

Streptomycin produces serious vestibular disturbances and sometimes deafness after prolonged treatment and less serious toxic symptoms such as nausea and vomiting make it an unpopular drug with patients.

Streptomycin is one of the most active agents in use against tubercle bacilli, and good results have been obtained in tuberculous meningitis and in acute, generalized or miliary tuberculosis. The main difficulty of streptomycin therapy in tuberculosis and in other diseases is the emergence of streptomycin-resistant strains. For this reason its use is practically restricted to the treatment of tuberculosis, and then only in combination with drugs such as *para*-aminosalicylate (PAS) or isoniazid, which prevent the emergence of resistant strains.

Streptomycin is a member of a family of antibiotics, the aminoglycosides, which includes among others the important agents *neomycin, gentamicin, amikacin* and *tobramycin*. Broadly speaking, these agents have the same spectrum of activity as streptomycin, but are more reliably active against infections with Gram-negative bacilli. The toxic effects of these agents are similar to those of streptomycin; neomycin, however, is too toxic for systemic use and is used locally or by mouth in intestinal infections as, like all the members of this family, it is not absorbed from the gut. Gentamicin, tobramycin and amikacin are valuable for the treatment of resistant Gram-negative infections including *Pseudomonas aeruginosa*.

Chloramphenicol

Chloramphenicol, also produced by some strains of streptomyces, is now produced synthetically. It is active against the Gram-positive cocci, Gram-negative bacilli, the organism of relapsing fever, the rickettsiae and some of the larger viruses. The rickettsiae, a group of organisms producing typhus and related infections, respond to treatment with chloramphenicol. Other diseases which respond are psittacosis and atypical virus pneumonia.

Chloramphenicol has the advantage of being absorbed from the gut and for many years has been the drug of choice for the treatment of enteric fever. The main limitation to its use is its liability to cause blood dyscrasias, in particular a fatal aplastic anaemia. For this reason it is restricted in practice to the treatment of certain severe, life-threatening infections.

The tetracyclines

Important broad-spectrum antibiotics in current use are the tetracyclines (tetracycline, oxytetracycline, chlortetracycline and others). These are all chemical derivatives of the core substance tetracycline and all have similar antibacterial activity and toxic effects.

Chlortetracycline. This antibiotic is produced by another strain of *Streptomyces.* It is well absorbed by mouth and the oral preparations available are stable when kept at room temperature. Injection solutions are less stable and should be freshly prepared. It is active against the Gram-negative bacilli and the Gram-positive and Gram-negative cocci. Certain Gram-negative bacilli such as the *Proteus, Klebsiella* and *Pseudomonas* groups are, however, relatively resistant.

Broad-spectrum antimicrobials

Drugs such as chloramphenicol, the tetracyclines and ampicillin have a wide range of antibacterial action, so that their administration inhibits the growth of both pathogenic and non-pathogenic organisms which are normally present on the healthy mucous membranes. These non-pathogens play a complex important part in the metabolism of the body. The bacterial flora of the gut and respiratory tract is profoundly altered after giving ampicillin, chloromycetin and chlortetracycline, and this change produces deleterious effects. The normal flora is liable to be replaced by antibiotic-resistant strains of species not normally found in these sites or only normally present in small numbers. For example, the gut flora may become overwhelmed by tetracycline-resistant staphylococci and the patient suffers the acute diarrhoeal disease of staphylococcal enterocolitis as a result, or the fungus *Candida albicans* may run riot in the gut or respiratory tract. In addition there may be vitamin B deficiency associated with the destruction of intestinal bacteria, which produces symptoms of vulval and anal irritation, and there may be vesiculopapular eruptions on the mucous membranes.

Erythromycin, lincomycin, clindamycin

These three antibiotics resemble each other in their action against Gram-positive organisms, particularly staphylococci, streptococci and pneumococci. Lincomycin and clindamycin are chemically closely related to each other but not to erythromycin. Despite the similarities there are important differences in the range of action against bacteria. Chief amongst these is that lincomycin and clindamycin are the most active drugs available for the treatment of infections caused by the anaerobic, non-sporing, *Bacteroides* group of organisms. In addition these two related drugs have the valuable property of being, to some degree, concentrated in bone and are therefore suitable for treating bone infections caused by bacteria which are sensitive to them.

Metronidazole

Metronidazole, was once regarded solely as an antiparasitic agent, widely used in the treatment of *Trichomonas* and certain gut infestations, but is now known to be effective in the treatment of anaerobic infections including those due to *Bacteroides* sp. Its use prophylactically before bowel surgery has considerably reduced the incidence of infection.

ANTIFUNGAL AGENTS

Most important antibiotics are produced by fungi, and it is understandable that fungi should be resistant to their effects. There are, however, a few substances that are effective in the treatment of certain human fungus infections. At present the most important of these are nystatin, amphotericin B, flucytosine and griseofulvin.

Nystatin, an almost completely insoluble antibiotic, is effective in the local treatment of moniliasis (infection with *Candida albicans*). It is too insoluble to be injected and it is not absorbed from the intestine, so that its use is restricted to local accessible infection of the mouth, gut and vagina.

Amphotericin B is a soluble, but fairly toxic, antibiotic active against *C. albicans* and a number of other fungi causing systemic infections. On account of its toxicity its use is very largely restricted to the treatment of serious systemic fungal infections.

Flucytosine is absorbed from the intestinal tract and has been used successfully in the treatment of systemic fungal infections due to *C. albicans* and certain other yeast-like fungi.

Griseofulvin is an antibiotic active against the fungi that cause ringworm. It is incorporated and excreted in the skin, thus being of special value in the treatment of fungus infections of difficult skin areas such as the hair and nails.

LIMITATIONS OF ANTIMICROBIAL CHEMOTHERAPY

The administration of almost any drug carries an element of risk to the patient. Inappropriate, inadequate or excessive dosage or an incomplete course of an antibiotic are all likely to have an adverse effect. It is as important for the correct dose to be prescribed and given as it it to select the most appropriate antibiotic to treat an infection.

Too great a concentration of certain antibiotics may have a serious toxic effect such as permanent renal damage or deafness. To reduce this risk, blood (serum) antibiotic levels should be monitored by laboratory assay at intervals during treatment and the dosage adjusted as necessary.

An inadequate dose or incomplete course of antibiotic may fail to cure the patient because the amount of the drug absorbed into the tissues is insufficient to combat the invading bacteria; there may then be a relapse, e.g. recurring streptococcal tonsilitis. Another effect of inadequate treatment is that sensitive organisms are destroyed but any survivors are likely to become antibiotic-resistant. This effect is produced, for example, by the indiscriminate application of topical antibiotics to superficial skin lesions, pressure sores and ulcers. Resistant bacteria develop, are transmitted to other patients, and cause an outbreak of infection which is very difficult to cure or control. For this reason many hospitals restrict the use of topical antibiotics as a matter of policy and suitable antiseptics are preferred for the treatment of most superficial infections.

More antibiotic substances are rapidly being discovered, and it is becoming apparent that these substances, which are so powerful, have disadvantages as well as advantages. Too little is yet known of the relationship between the metabolism of the normal bacterial flora and the host metabolism, and the administration of one antibiotic may produce an incidental effect on the other organisms on the mucous membranes, with the development of an antibiotic-fast strain of bacteria which may last for many bacterial generations.

To sum up, it is true to say that there are antibiotics now available to deal with the whole pathogenic bacterial kingdom, and the future course of bacterial disease may well depend upon the proper use of the right one.

Antibiotic treatment cannot replace antiserum treatment in the toxaemia such as tetanus, gas gangrene and diphtheria; the two lines of treatment must go together. The antibiotic inhibits the growth of the organism, but does not neutralize the preformed toxin. The treatment of the virus diseases, however, other than the diseases caused by the large ones, is another matter. Their position, intracellular and out of reach of the tissue fluids, and the fact that their metabolism is so intimately bound up with that of the host metabolism, has so far made many of them immune to available chemotherapeutic agents and antibiotics.

Summary of Antimicrobial Agents

Antimicrobial Chemotherapeutic Agent	Indications for Use	Notes
PENICILLINS		
Benzyl penicillin (Pen. G)	Gram-positive bacteria; Gram-negative cocci	Parenteral use only
Phenoxymethyl penicillin (Pen. V)	For mild infections as above	Oral only. Absorption variable
Methicillin	⎱ Effective against penicillinase-resistant staphylococci	Parenteral use
Flucloxacillin	⎰	Parenteral or oral use
Ampicillin	⎱ Broad-spectrum activity: coliforms, *Proteus*, *Str. faecalis*, *Haemophilus influenzae*	Destroyed by penicillinase-producing staphylococci. May induce a skin rash
Amoxycillin	⎰ Many *Ps. aeruginosa* infections	May induce a skin rash
Carbenicillin	Specifically *Ps. aeruginosa* urinary tract infections	Oral only. Urinary tract activity only
Carfecillin	⎱	Parenteral use only
Azlocillin	⎰	
Mezlocillin	⎱ Broadly similar activity to carbenicillin but more effective weight for weight	
Ticarcillin	⎰	
Piperacillin		
CEPHALOSPORINS		
Cephaloridine	⎱ All have broad spectrum activity against Gram-positive and Gram-negative rods and penicillinase-producing staphylococci	Diuretics, especially frusemide, are prescribed with great caution because of the risk of renal failure
Cephalothin	⎰	May be painful injection: cephaloridine or cephalothin
Cephalexin	⎱	Oral, cephalexin; oral/parenteral, cephaloridine
Cephradine	⎰ Activity against Gram-negatives greater than above	Parenteral use only
Cefamandole		
Cefoxitin		
Cefuroxime		

Erythromycin	All are active against staphylococci, streptococci, pneumococci, *Bacteroides*	If erythromycin is the sole antibiotic used *Staph. aureus* may develop resistance
Lincomycin Clindamycin	} Bone infections	Lincomycin may cause intestinal upset; give with food Clindamycin: colitis is a rare toxic effect
Fusidic acid	*Staph. aureus* infections	May cause intestinal upset
Tetracycline	Broad-spectrum activity Bacteriostatic	May cause nausea; give in milk Contra-indicated in renal failure and for children (teeth) Toxic effect: diarrhoea
Chloramphenicol	Enteric fever. *H. influenzae* meningitis. Topical eye medications	Toxic effect: aplastic anaemia
Sulphonamides Trimethoprim Co-trimoxazole (Septrin)	Wide spectrum of activity Mostly active against Gram-negative organisms Broad spectrum: streptococci, staphylococci, all Gram-negatives except *Ps. aeruginosa*	May cause a rash/crystalluria. Always used in combination Used alone mainly for urinary tract infections Combination of a sulphonamide and trimethoprim May cause nausea
AMINOGLYCOSIDES Streptomycin Kanamycin Neomycin Gentamicin Amikacin Tobramycin	Tuberculosis Gut 'sterilization': not absorbed from the bowel } Broad spectrum: serious Gram-negative infections, including *Pseudomonas* spp.	Toxic effect: 8th cranial nerve damage (vestibular) Toxic effect: 8th cranial nerve damage (auditory) Too toxic for systemic use. Oral/topical Toxic effect: 8th cranial nerve damage (vestibular) Laboratory assay of serum levels usually ordered to control dosage
Nitrofurantoin Nalidixic acid	Gram-negative urinary tract infections only	May cause nausea

Antimicrobial Chemotherapeutic Agent	Indications for Use	Notes
ANTI-TUBERCULOUS THERAPY		
Streptomycin[1] (see above)	Long term therapy is given in combination,	PAS: large capsule
Isoniazid[2]	e.g. 1+2+5/3 for one to two months	Rifampicin causes red urine, tears, sputum. Given
Para-aminosalicylate[3] (PAS)	then 2+5/3+4 for 18 months or	before food for better absorption. May cause a
Rifampicin[4]	4+2+5 all given orally	rash or intestinal upset. Antibodies develop after
Ethambutol[5]		the course so no second course can be given.
Thiacetazone[6]		Thiacetazone successfully used in the developing countries
Metronidazole	*Bacteroides* infections. Anti-parasitic agent	
ANTI-FUNGAL THERAPY		
Nystatin	Moniliasis of mouth, gut, vagina	Insoluble, topical application
Amphotericin B	Serious systemic fungal infections	Very toxic
Flucytosine	Serious systemic fungal infections	Less toxic
Griseofulvin	Ringworm and dermatophytes	Oral use
ANTI-VIRAL THERAPY		
Cytosine arabinoside	Herpesvirus infections	Parenteral
Idoxuridine	Herpesvirus infections	Topical application of limited value
Methisazone	Smallpox contacts	Side effect: nausea. Given only to high-risk, non-immune contacts for very short-term passive immunity

7 Sterilization and Disinfection

Just as organisms vary in the factors and conditions necessary for their growth, so they differ in their response to adverse conditions both physical and chemical. Some are killed easily by brief exposure to a relatively low temperature, e.g. typhoid bacilli; some, like *Clostridium tetani*, still live after prolonged exposure to a high temperature. Some organisms, particularly viruses, are relatively susceptible to one type of killing agent, but resistant to another. The sensitivity of an organism to a killing agent is known as the organism's innate susceptibility and it depends upon many factors.

The bacterial kingdom with which the medical microbiologist is concerned can be divided into two parts, this division being based on the Gram stain, as described in Chapter 8. The ability to retain the dye which is shown by the Gram-positive organisms obviously reflects a very different chemical constitution, and the Gram-positive organisms are different in their response to killing agents from the Gram-negative organisms. The Gram-positive group includes a subgroup of organisms which are difficult to kill and which are at the same time highly dangerous to man in certain circumstances. They are the spore-bearing group to which *Cl. tetani, Bacillus anthracis* and *Cl. botulinum* belong.

It is important to define the two terms which refer to the killing of microbes:

Sterilization. The destruction or removal of all microorganisms including spores. Usually by heat.

Disinfection. The reduction in numbers or destruction of harmful micro-organisms not usually including bacterial spores. Usually by chemical agents or some form of wet heat.

When assessing a killing agent, the innate susceptibility of the organism it is desired to kill must be considered, and there are other factors which will influence the action of the killing agent:

1. The time necessary for action.
2. The concentration of killing agent.
3. The optimum acidity, or alkalinity for activity of killing agent.
4. The optimum temperature.
5. The numbers of organisms present.
6. The physical state of the material from which it is necessary to remove the bacteria; protein, blood, pus, mucus and dirt act as a protective coat for the bacteria and limit the action of killing agents.
7. Direct contact between all surfaces of the object to be sterilized and the killing agent. Air bubbles in tubing will protect bacteria from steam or chemicals.
8. Antagonistic substances neutralizing the activity of the killing agent.
9. Impurities diluting the agent.
10. Inactivation of the agent by time.

THE CHOICE OF KILLING AGENTS

Choosing a killing agent or bactericide for a particular purpose is a relatively simple matter if the contaminating organism is known.

● If a child has impetigo due to haemolytic *Streptococcus* the infecting organism must be removed from his toys by some killing agent before the toys are played with by other children. The innate susceptibility of the haemolytic *Streptococcus* is known and the choice of killing agent is wide, the limiting factor being the size and type of material to be disinfected. The particular process is designed to remove the *Streptococcus,* which is a relatively susceptible organism; it will not necessarily remove other more resistant organisms which may be present on the toys, that is to say the toys are not necessarily made sterile or free from all organisms.

● The choice of the killing agent to be used against the *Streptococcus* on the skin of the patient, however, is governed by another limiting factor. The agent must be poisonous to the pathogenic organism in concentrations which are not harmful to the patient.

Materials or instruments which are to be introduced into the body, or which touch sites from which pathogenic organisms can get into the body, must be made completely sterile and free from all organisms. Dust contains large numbers of organisms which, being light and small, can be wafted in air currents for long distances. It is not possible to know what organisms are present unless extensive bacteriological tests are done. To be on the safe side, therefore, all materials and instruments to be introduced into the body must be submitted to rigorous sterilizing techniques. The choice of killing agents in these cases is limited to those physical or chemical agents which will kill the most resistant organisms. Sterilization techniques should be checked at frequent intervals (see Appendix I).

DEATH OF MICRO-ORGANISMS

Contact between a sterilizing agent and micro-organisms effects a reduction in the number of organisms; most die, a few survive. If the survivors are exposed to continuous contact with the sterilizing agent virtually all of them will be killed in time. Only a minute percentage of very resistant organisms will survive, perhaps 1 in 10^6 with a marginally acceptable sterilizing method or only 1 in 10^{50} with an efficient method such as autoclaving. The percentage of surviving organisms and the time taken to kill them is dependent on several factors: the number of organisms initially present, the efficiency and reliability of the sterilizing agent and the correct application. A comparatively inefficient agent will take a long time to reduce the number of survivors to an acceptable risk level.

CLEANING

If the number of organisms present affects sterilizing time and efficiency it is clearly of practical importance to reduce the numbers as far as possible before attempting to apply any method of sterilization. It is also essential to remove organic material which will protect bacteria against the action of physical or chemical agents by preventing direct contact.

Careful washing of skin, equipment or instruments in plenty of hot water with soap or detergent does not remove all bacteria but it does remove grease and dirt which protect bacteria, and it does effectively reduce the numbers of bacteria. Whenever possible, running water not hot enough to coagulate protein, i.e. $< 60°C$, should be used so that bacteria are not simply transferred to the water in the washing bowl. Where there are considerable quantities of equipment to be cleaned, e.g. central sterilizing or central food service departments, automatic jet or deluge washing machines are used to give the most effective wash in a reasonable time.

The development of ultrasonic cleaning equipment for use in hospitals has improved standards of cleaning delicate

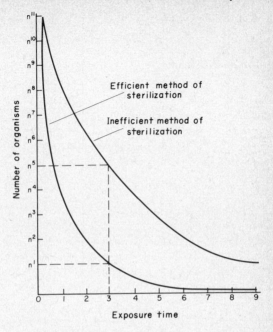

Fig. 17. With the same exposure time, e.g. 3, an efficient sterilizing method reduces the number of organisms from n^{11} to n^1. An inefficient sterilizing method only reduces the number from n^{11} to n^5.

instruments with ridges and awkward crevices. The source of energy is very high frequency sound waves generated in the base of a tank of water to which detergent is added, and in which baskets or racks of instruments are submerged. The ensuing shock waves dislodge dirt on the submerged instruments. These are subsequently rinsed and dried. The effect of shock waves can be shown by placing a piece of foil on the surface of the water; when the tank is activated pin holes rapidly appear in the foil.

STERILIZATION

Methods of sterilization

Heat	Dry	Direct application—Incineration
		Hot air oven
		Infra-red conveyor
	Moist	Steam under pressure—121°C at 1.05 kg/cm²
		134°C at 2.1 kg/cm²
		Low temperature steam—80°C
		(see Gases)
Chemicals	Gases	L.T.S. & formaldehyde
		Ethylene oxide
	Liquids	Glutaraldehyde
Radiation		Ionizing radiation—Gamma rays
		—Particulate high-energy electrons
Filtration		

HEAT

Heat resistance of organisms. Different species of micro-organisms vary greatly in their ability to withstand heat. Some such as the gonococcus are very sensitive and will be killed by a few minutes' exposure at 47°C. The majority die after 2–30 min exposure to 50–70°C moist heat. Some, for example *Streptococcus faecalis,* are more resistant and a few with the ability to form spores are very resistant. Since these spore-forming organisms are dangerous to a patient who has sustained an injury or surgery resulting in muscle tissue lacking an adequate oxygen supply, all hospital sterilization procedures aim to kill spore-forming bacteria. Procedures which destroy organisms except the spore formers are described as disinfection or sanitization procedures.

Time/temperature relationship. Destruction of micro-organisms by heat is achieved by rapid coagulation of the cell protein with moist heat or by a much slower process of oxidization with dry heat. In either case it is necessary to apply the minimum temperature known to kill, and to maintain this temperature for a definite length of time since the cell wall affords some protection and death is not instantaneous. If the temperature is raised, the exposure time can be decreased. For example a standard time/temperature ratio for moist heat is 121°C for 15 min, if the temperature is raised to 134°C the time required for sterilization is decreased to 3 min (Medical Research Council (1959). Sterilization by steam under increased pressure. *Lancet*, **i**, 425).

Dry heat

Dry heat is transferred from source to load by conduction or radiation. High temperatures and comparatively long exposure times are required. These two facts explain why it is not a suitable sterilizing agent for fabrics and dressings which are poor uneven conductors and ruined by excessive heat. It is, however, the method of choice for fine metal cannulae such as lumbar puncture needles and for all glass syringes since these can then be sterilized with a stilette or plunger in position, heating by conduction ensuring sterilization of the inside. The need for this has lessened since the general use of disposable syringes, but this method is of use for sterilization of some ophthalmic instruments liable to damage by moist heat. Dry heat is also used to sterilize oily pharmaceutical preparations and powders. Sterilizing exposure time is always measured from the point at which the centre of the load attains the required sterilizing (holding) temperature. This will vary according to the size of the load and the type of material being processed, and necessitates careful control and testing of the apparatus (Appendix I).

Direct-application flame. Incineration is the safest method of sterilizing and disposing of infected dressings.

Laboratory wire loops used for transferring bacteria and inoculating media are sterilized by heating to redness in a Bunsen burner flame.

Hot air oven. The standard temperature/time ratio is 160°C for 60 min. The total cycle time is considerably longer since it includes the time required for the whole load to attain 160°C prior to exposure time, plus the time required for the load to cool down after sterilization. Hot air ovens used for sterilization must contain a fan to ensure air circulation and thus an even temperature at all levels within the oven.

Infra-red conveyor sterilizer. The standard sterilizing temperature/time ratio is 180°C for 7½ mins holding time. Metal instruments, needles and glass syringes in containers are placed on a conveyor belt forming the floor of a tunnel, in the roof of which is a series of infra-red heating elements. The speed of the conveyor is regulated to allow heating of the load by radiation and conduction to 180°C and maintenance at this temperature for 7½ mins.

This apparatus is larger and more difficult to regulate than a hot air oven.

Moist heat

Relatively low temperatures will destroy micro-organisms in the presence of moisture, 121°C for 15 min exposure to steam under pressure is equivalent in effect to 160°C for 60 min exposure to dry heat. Temperatures greater than 100°C are required for reliable sterilization in reasonable. time. Pasteurization, boiling, cystoscope 'pasteurization' and UCT tyndallization (a discontinuous steaming process used in the laboratory) do not kill all spore-forming bacteria and are methods of disinfection not sterilization.

Steam under pressure. Steam under pressure as used in autoclaves has physical properties which allow rapid penetration of porous objects and fabrics as well as sterilization of instruments and solid objects. Temperatures greater than the 121°C for 15 min required to kill spores can be readily obtained and this is the commonest and most reliable method of sterilizing dressings, linen, instruments and equipment in hospitals.

PHYSICAL PROPERTIES OF STEAM

Latent heat. The temperature of 1 g of water is raised 1°C by 4.2J (1 calorie). 336J (80 calories) are required to raise 1 g of water at 20°C to boiling point (100°C). A further 2200J (524 calories are required to turn 1 g of water at 100°C to 1 g of steam at the same temperature. These 2200J (524 calories) are stored in the steam as latent heat. Latent heat is transferred to an object to be sterilized by the steam condensing on the cooler surface as a film of moisture, releasing and transferring the heat instantaneously. This process continues until the object to be sterilized is at the same temperature as the steam; then, sterilization exposure time starts. Steam is able to penetrate porous materials very rapidly provided that it is not impeded by unsuitable wrappings or air trapped within fabrics or hollow instruments.

Air/steam mixture. Air and steam mix by slow diffusion. When steam is introduced into a vessel such as an autoclave which already contains air, the air being heavier (density 0.12) and cooler than steam (density 0.07) will remain at the bottom of the vessel where the temperature will be significantly lower.

The removal of air from an autoclave during the sterilizing cycle is important for two reasons. Air left in the centre of a pack of linen or in a narrow cannula such as a catheter will prevent the steam from coming into direct contact with the centre towels or the lumen in the centre of the catheter. Failure to contact means failure to sterilize.

Secondly, air mixed with steam reduces the temperature of the steam. For example, when a standard pressure of 1.7 kg/cm² (25 lb/in²) of steam is used in an autoclave the relationship of air discharge/temperature/time required for sterilization is shown in the following table:

Air discharge	Temperature	Sterilizing time
None	115°C	Spores are not killed
1/3	121°C	15 min
2/3	126°C	12 min
Complete	132°C	3 min

Steam pressure. Increasing the pressure of steam in the absence of air increases the temperature. The temperature of steam at 1.05 kg/cm² (15 lb/in²) is 121°C, at 1.35 kg/cm² (20 lb/in²) is 126°C and at 2.1 kg/cm² (30 lb/in²) is 134°C.

Quality of steam. Steam used for sterilizing must have exact characteristics and is described as dry, saturated steam at phase boundary between vapour and water.

Autoclaves
Three types of autoclave are widely used in hospitals:

1. Downward displacement for unwrapped instruments.
2. Fluid and laboratory.
3. High vacuum.

They vary from comparatively simple vessels with manually controlled steam inlet and outlet, to highly complex fully automatic machines. Each has a particular function and is used to sterilize a different type of load. All consist basically of a chamber with air-tight doors, constructed to withstand high internal pressures and equipped with a safety valve, controlled steam inlet, chamber drain, thermometer in the outlet drain line, temperature and steam pressure recorders.

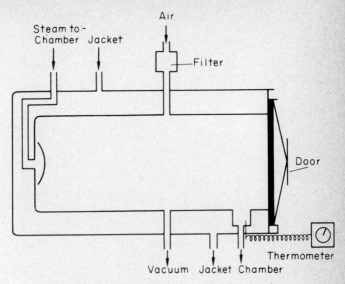

Fig. 18. Diagrammatic representation of an autoclave.

Downward displacement autoclave. Steam enters the upper part of the chamber and being lighter, displaces air downwards and out of the drain line. A thermostatic steam trap controls the air and condensate discharge. An autoclave of this type is suitable for unwrapped instrument and surface sterilization. It will not sterilize packs or tubing since air would be trapped within them, preventing steam penetration; nor is it suitable for fabrics and paper which would be wet at the end of the cycle. It is important to load the autoclave carefully to facilitate air displacement and free steam circulation.

Autoclaves for fluids and laboratory use. These autoclaves operate on the same principle as the displacement type but usually can be operated at a variety of steam pressures thus allowing a wider range of temperature settings. They often

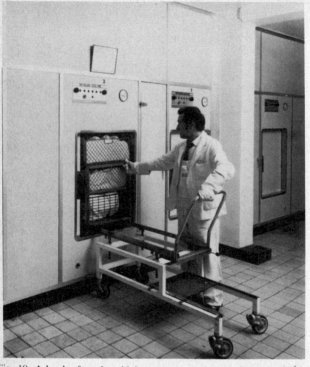

Fig. 19. A bank of modern high vacuum autoclaves being unloaded in a Central Sterile Department. *(British Sterilizer Co. Ltd.)*

have a slow exhaust cycle to prevent fluids from 'boiling' over or bottles from exploding. Some models have a post-sterilization water cooling cycle which shortens the total time by cooling the outside of the sterilized bottles and allows the operator to open the autoclave door at the end of the cycle without risk of cooler room air in contact with extremely hot bottles causing explosion and injury. They should be fitted with an inner safety door for the same reason.

Bottles of fluids prepared for sterilization should be three quarters filled, and capped. Sterilization exposure time depends on the size of the container. For example at 121°C a 500 ml bottle requires 24 min while a 2000 ml bottle requires 40 min exposure.

High vacuum autoclaves. These are very complex, automatically operated, jacketed autoclaves designed for efficient, fast sterilization of air-trapping loads such as packs of fabrics, dressings and instruments, limited lengths of tubing and hollow equipment. The complexity of the machines and the critical importance of air displacement from the load make regular skilled maintenance and testing essential to safe sterilizing practice (Appendix I).

High vacuum autoclave cycle. The autoclave is loaded and the automatic cycle, which in modern machines includes door closure, is started. Air contained within the chamber, within the packs and their contents, is pumped out through the outlet drain, i.e. a vacuum is drawn to reduce the pressure from 100 kPa (760 mm Hg) (atmospheric) to less than 2.5 kPa (20 mm Hg) in the chamber. A minute amount of air (<3%) remains. Air is much more easily and quickly displaced from the space surrounding the load than from the centre of the packs and their contents. It follows that if the autoclave is loaded with only one or two small packs, there is a danger that the residual air will be concentrated in the centre of the packs where it will prevent steam penetration and therefore sterilization. To increase efficiency and to safeguard against this 'small load phenomenon' a steam pulsing phase has been added to most high vacuum autoclave cycles. At the beginning of the sterilizing phase, steam under pressure is pulsed into, and withdrawn from, the chamber in a series of six rapid bursts to ensure movement and diffusion of any remaining air. Because of the vacuum, steam is immediately able to penetrate to the centre of the packs and equipment. Sterilization exposure time (see page 75) is measured from the point at which the load attains the same temperature as the steam, usually 134°C for 3 min. A second or post-sterilizing vacuum is drawn to remove the steam from the load. Filtered sterile air is then allowed into the chamber to replace the vacuum, maintaining the sterility of the load.

A porous load autoclave is surrounded by a steam insulating jacket which is not connected to the chamber. Its function is to prevent heat loss during the sterilizing phase and to assist in the rapid drying of the load which occurs during the post-sterilizing vacuum, and vacuum breaking phases. The steam supply to the jacket is not normally turned off, the jacket is therefore constantly at sterilizing temperature. Excessive drying of the load, damage to fabrics, and sterilizing failures due to the superheated steam will occur if the load is held in the autoclave for any length of time prior to starting the cycle.

Low temperature steam. This is a method of killing all vegetative organisms and most spores present on heat sensitive equipment such as endoscopes when combined with a chemical vapour, *formaldehyde*. A high vacuum autoclave is modified to admit steam at subatmospheric pressure so that the temperature in the chamber does not rise above 80°C. Exposure times of 30 min to 2 h are recommended, varying according to the material to be processed.

The disadvantages of the gas are that it has a pungent smell, is irritant to eyes, skin and mucous membranes, and has poor properties of penetration and diffusion into fabrics or narrow tubes such as catheters. Materials must also be packed in a way that allows the vapour to penetrate, and they require lengthy 'airing' to remove the toxic gases afterwards.

Formaldehyde catheter 'sterilizing' ovens are unreliable and unsatisfactory; they should not be used (Department of Health and Social Security recommendation 1969).

Ethylene oxide sterilization may be used for sterilization of even more heat-sensitive materials requiring temperatures of 45–60°C (usually 55°C) and a holding time of 2 to 4 h. Ethylene oxide is a highly reactive colourless liquid with a boiling point of 10.7°C which is used in a gaseous state for sterilization of heat-sensitive materials. It has been used for many years to preserve foodstuffs and as an insecticide but only comparatively recently for medical purposes. The gas can be used at comparatively low temperatures, it does not corrode or damage a wide range of materials and, though much slower and less reliable than moist or dry heat, is a means of sterilizing equipment which would be ruined by both heat and ionizing radiation. The sterilizing process should be under skilled supervision since the efficiency of this agent is dependent on the correct balance of many interrelated factors.

1. Ethylene oxide penetrates and diffuses readily through porous loads, rubber and most plastics. A few plastics are adversely affected and acquire internal stresses after processing causing them to break in use. Penetration time, and therefore total sterilizing cycle time, varies according to the wrapping material as well as to the item contained in it. For example polyvinyl chloride films, aluminium laminates and films greater than 0.08 mm thick are relatively impermeable, penetration of Cellophane wrap is slow, but polythene and paper are easily and quickly permeated. Some metals (magnesium, zinc, tin) should not be exposed to the gas since they combine with ethylene oxide to form a sticky gel.

2. An effective cleaning process is of the greatest importance. As in every other sterilizing method, organic substances particularly proteins will prevent the essential contact between bacteria and the sterilizing agent. Bacteria suspended in salt solution are incorporated into the crystalline deposit on evaporation. This crystalline deposit

is able to protect the bacteria from ethylene oxide and prevents their destruction. Both dirt and salt crystals remaining on equipment prevent sterilization by ethylene oxide.

3. It is thought that the gas has to be in solution on the bacterial cell surface to enable it to penetrate the cell wall and destroy the bacterium. Therefore both an adequate concentration of gas and sufficient moisture content throughout the load are also vital factors in achieving sterilization. It is important to avoid hot dry storage rooms and storage cupboards, the humidity in the preparation and packing areas should not be less than 50%. If the sterilizing load is a mixed one, containing perhaps two different plastics, metal, paper and rubber it is very difficult to ensure an even and adequate distribution of both gas and moisture since the materials vary in density and moisture-retaining properties. It is even more difficult to establish a satisfactory but practical testing method.

4. Modern apparatus is designed to remove air from the loaded ethylene oxide sterilizer before the humidified gas is introduced. This facilitates even penetration of the load, eliminates the possibility of an explosive air/gas mixture and allows the use of pure ethylene oxide. Other apparatus which does not have a vacuum cycle commonly utilizes a mixture of 10% ethylene oxide and 90% of an inert gas such as carbon dioxide or freon to avoid the risk of an explosion.

5. Sterilization can be achieved at room temperature but requires a very long exposure time. The recommended gas concentration in and on the load is between 450 and 900 mg/litre.

6. Controlled conditions are essential for load packing, penetration and sterilization. They are equally essential for the safety of patients and staff handling packs and equipment after sterilization. Ethylene oxide takes time to

diffuse out from materials, particularly rubber and plastics. The airing time required, even when a post vacuum is used, may be as long as 48 h. Gas retained in equipment held in contact with the skin or mucous membrane will produce irritation and blistering.

Although the toxicity is defined as low and reversible the effects are unpleasant and in addition to adequate airing time, other safety measures such as good ventilation, correctly installed machine exhaust lines, and regular maintenance to detect and prevent leaks is necessary.

Liquid chemicals
Glutaraldehyde (see page 96). This compound is said to be able to be used for sterilization of heat-sensitive items such as fibre-optic endoscopes if they are immersed for up to three hours. This is rarely practicable and a shorter immersion leading to disinfection is usually all that is achieved.

RADIATION

Ionizing radiation
The scientific exploration and development of the peaceful uses of atomic energy is a twentieth century achievement which has made considerable contributions to the advancement of medical technology. In the field of sterilization, particularly in the United Kingdom, a very reliable means of sterilizing thermolabile (heat-sensitive) materials has become commercially available at a reasonable cost. The size of the plant, the cost of the source, and the statutory safeguards required in the handling of radioactive materials determine that the method is nationally and commercially, rather than hospital centred.

Sources. Two sources of ionizing radiation are now used:

1. Gamma rays from the radio-isotope cobalt 60.

2. Particulate high-energy electrons from a linear accelerator.
Gamma rays have the greater power of penetration so that while standard medical packs for gamma irradiation are up to 30 cm thick, those for electron beam processing are usually single, small items. Penetration in both cases is dependent on the density of the material being processed; standard packs allow for mixed contents.

The plants are fully automatic to avoid exposing operators to ionizing radiation. Conveyor belts carry standard sized packs, at standard speed, past the source so that each pack receives a measured dose. It is usual for packs to be automatically turned and irradiated from more than one side in such a plant.

Dose. The International Atomic Energy Agency of the United Nations Working Party's recommended code of practice for radiation sterilization (1967), covers many aspects of packaging and plant control including the dose requirement. In the United Kingdom and several other countries a radiation sterilization dose of 2.5 Mrad has been in use for medical disposable products for over fifteen years. At this dosage it is important that articles to be sterilized are, as far as possible, free from living virus particles. This is because the dosage of radiation required to kill micro-organisms is inversely proportional to the particle size, i.e. a larger dose of radiation is required to kill a small virus particle than to kill a large bacterial particle.

A rad is a unit of measurement of energy absorbed from radiation by the matter through which it passes. 1 rad involves the liberation of 100 ergs of energy into each gram. In practical terms this means that the rise in temperature during sterilization is only a few degrees C. 1 Mrad = 1 million rads.

Suitable materials. Ionizing radiation never induces radioactivity in the materials being processed but it may induce chemical change in some materials making them temporarily or permanently unstable and therefore unsuited to the process. Teflon (PTFE) and rubbers are examples of materials in which permanent damage is or may be induced. The following can usually be safely irradiated for single use: nylon, polythene, polystyrene, PVC, Terylene, cotton, paper and wool products. Sugar, which turns pink but reverts, is an example of temporary instability.

Ability to sterilize the increasing numbers of disposable plastic items such as syringes and catheters which will not withstand heat sterilization, and 'sharps' such as hypodermic needles and scalpel blades is of great value. These can now be packed before sterilization in individual sealed aluminium foil or plastic packs contained in an outer carbon carton ready for dispatch, avoiding any handling and possible recontamination after sterilization.

FILTRATION

Pharmaceutical fluids and laboratory media which would be damaged by heat, ionizing radiation or chemicals are passed through filters to remove micro-organisms. The filters vary in material and design, e.g. porous membranes such as asbestos or glass fibre.

Air free from micro-organisms which may cause infection is required in operating theatres and other units for the protection of patients at high risk from infection. It is also a requirement where air is drawn into a sterile field such as the air inlet of an intravenous infusion set or an autoclave at the end of the sterilizing cycle. Protection from respiratory organisms may be achieved by the use of an efficient mask or a specially designed filter, e.g. a William's filter fitted into the circuit of a respirator.

Although the filters mentioned range from a wisp of cotton wool to a high efficiency particulate air filter (99.9% efficiency, 1 to 5 μm), if each is examined under a microscope the holes or the spaces between the fibres will be seen to be very much larger than the particles which they trap. Air passing through a filter induces a positive static charge in the fibres to which particles are attracted and held. If the fibres become moist the charge is earthed and the particles released, that is, a wet filter, e.g. a wet mask, allows organisms to pass through it.

DISINFECTION

Methods of disinfection

Moist heat	Pasteurization
	Boiling water
	Low temperatures (subatmospheric) steam
Gases	Formaldehyde
Chemical agents	Halogens
	Phenolics
	Diguanides
	Quaternary ammonium compounds $\pm$ Diguanides
	Alcohols
	Aldehydes

Disinfection (see page 70) is not so precise an activity as sterilization. It should be realized by all involved that it does not mean sterilization, and so should only be used for situations where an overall reduction of micro-organisms is sufficient for safety of patients and staff. There are occasions when it is used to treat heat-sensitive items as the nearest approach possible to sterility, but the difference must still be acknowledged.

Methods of disinfection are shown in the table above, but should always be preceded by a thorough cleaning of the item to be disinfected. Cleaning with a detergent and hot water will remove the majority of micro-organisms present.

MOIST HEAT

Pasteurization. Pasteurization is the method of heat treatment of milk to make it safe for human consumption by removal of pathogenic bacteria such as *Brucella, Streptococcus pyogenes,* or tubercle bacilli which are frequently carried in milk; it is not a method of sterilization, but those organisms which remain after pasteurization are harmless when ingested.

There are two methods of pasteurization in common use in this country. The Holder process entails raising the temperature of the milk to 62°C, keeping it there for 30 min, then cooling quickly to 13°C or below. The Flash method keeps the milk at a temperature of not less than 74°C for 3–5 sec followed by cooling quickly to 13°C or below. Pasteurization removes the pathogenic bacteria in milk, with the advantage over boiling that it does not alter the taste unpleasantly. In both processes the rapid cooling is important for the keeping properties of the milk as it minimizes multiplication of surviving non-pathogenic bacteria.

Pasteurization of cystoscopes. Many cystoscopes would be damaged by high temperatures and are disinfected, not sterilized, for this reason. The term pasteurization should only be applied to the processing of milk described above but it is colloquially used to describe the total immersion of instruments such as cystoscopes in a water bath at 75°C for 10 min to destroy non-sporing organisms.

Boiling. Total immersion in boiling water (100°C) for 5 min will kill most pathogenic organisms and is the most reliable method of disinfecting (not sterilizing) instruments and apparatus. It is important to ensure that all items are completely submerged and that no air is trapped within bowls or hollow instruments. No destructive agent, physical or chemical, is effective unless it is in direct contact with all surfaces. Air has the effect of preventing contact and lowering temperature. The required 5 min exposure time is measured from the time when the water actually boils again after the last instruments have been immersed.

Two pairs of Cheatle's or transfer forceps are required for removing instruments or bowls from the boiler after processing. These should be stored in proximity to the boiler in sterile packets, for single-use only. If this is not possible they should be stored in a clear-soluble phenolic disinfectant and the solution should be changed daily, with forceps and container also being cleaned daily.

Low-temperature (subatmospheric) steam may be used for disinfection of some heat-sensitive materials. For sterilization formaldehyde would need to be added.

GASES

Formaldehyde
This gas is occasionally used for terminal room disinfection and as a means of disinfecting mechanical apparatus such as patient ventilators. Extreme care in removing all traces of the gas by neutralizing with ammonia followed by very thorough airing of equipment before use is essential to patient safety.

CHEMICAL AGENTS

There are a bewildering number of chemical preparations on the market. Very few of them are reliable *sterilizing agents* in the strengths and under the circumstances in which they are used in the home or in hospital. An *antiseptic* inhibits micro-organisms (i.e. prevents growth and multiplication). The term antiseptic is used of weaker and less toxic solutions which inhibit, and may kill. It is commonly used to describe applications to living tissue. *Germicide* is a newer word meaning a chemical capable of killing micro-organisms.

The suffix -*cide* indicates that an agent kills. Bactericides kill bacteria. Fungicides kill fungi.

The suffix -*stat* indicates that an agent prevents or inhibits growth.

No single preparation fulfills all requirements and all are less reliable than heat or radiation as sterilizing agents.

Too often the choice of chemical agent is a matter of whim or fashion which results in unjustifiable expense and inefficient practice. It is helpful if a committee such as a hospital control of infection committee which includes a pharmacist is responsible for advising on the selection and use of disinfectants, germicides and antiseptics. The aim of the committee should be to select efficient agents, to define the dilutions and exposure times appropriate to specific uses, and to limit the number of agents purchased. This 'disinfectant policy' should help rationalize the use of disinfectant solutions and enable staff to use the right solution for the right purpose.

Consideration should be given to these important factors when making an assessment:

1. The need: (*a*) Decontamination of inanimate objects such as floors, furniture, kitchen equipment, infected linen, medical and nursing equipment. (*b*) Decontamination of living tissue such as skin, wounds, eyes, body cavities.

2. Any known local conditions or problems, e.g. a high incidence of staphylococcal infection, a tuberculosis unit. Some organisms are very resistant to the action of chemical agents, e.g. *Pseudomonas aeruginosa*.

3. The efficiency of the agents, basing judgements on in-use tests (Kelsey & Maurer 1974), i.e. the performance in clean and dirty working situations (see Appendix II).

4. Safety for both patients and staff. Preferably chemicals which are neither irritant, toxic, nor corrosive.

5. The degree of hardness of the local water to be used for dilution purposes. This may affect the efficiency of the agent, as it seems that different disinfectants are affected by differences in pH.

6. Stability during storage and in use.

7. Time taken to act.

8. Any other problems produced by use, e.g. staining of bed and personal linen, corrosion of metal, sensitization.

9. Cost.

Guide lines for use should include reminders:

● Never use chemicals if more reliable methods are available.

● Cleaning is the first and most important step in chemical disinfection.

● Total surface contact is essential.

● Recommended strengths for specific purposes must be known and adhered to, e.g. clean and dirty situations.

● No agent acts instantaneously. Note the recommended exposure time.

● Equipment has to be rinsed after immersion in a chemical. It is very easy to recontaminate it at this stage unless sterile water, dishes and forceps are used.

● Antiseptics and ointments may themselves become contaminated by incorrect use, e.g. by placing a hand or swab on the top of a bottle or by dipping fingers into containers or ointment or cream. They vary in antimicrobial activity and are not effective against every type of organism which may be picked up and transferred by hands.

● Many materials cause inactivation of chemical disinfectants. These range from pus and blood through rubber and cellulose products to most manmade materials such as PVC and nylon. Inactivation is probably the main drawback to using chemical disinfectants.

The halogens—chlorine and iodine compounds

Iodine 2.5% in 70% alcohol is perhaps the most effective skin germicide but it is an irritant and may cause a severe reaction in a sensitive subject and has the further disadvantage of staining. The *iodophors,* e.g. providone-iodine (Betadine, Wescodyne), are combinations of iodine and non-ionic detergents. They have the good properties of iodine but are non-staining, much less toxic, and less irritant. The solutions contain a colour indicator which fades as the germicidal activity diminishes. They are used mainly for hand and skin disinfection.

Chlorine compounds such as chlorinated lime, and hypochlorites, are capable of liberating active chlorine. *Chlorinated lime* or domestic bleach is used for disinfecting drinking water, swimming baths, drains, etc. Since chlorine compounds are relatively easily inhibited by organic matter it is important to keep drain traps and overflows clean in addition to using the disinfectant. *Eusol* is a chlorinated lime and boric acid compound used for wound dressings and packs but is usually considered to be too irritant for irrigation purposes. *Dakin's solution* (surgical chlorinated soda solution BPC) and ESH (electrolytic sodium hypochlorite) are used for wound irrigation and dressings. Milton (1% sodium hypochlorite) is also commonly used to disinfect baby-bottles and for kitchen hygiene. Hypochlorites are effective against most viruses and are of great value where hepatitis viruses may be a danger.

Phenolic compounds

These are coal tar derivatives which have been in use in hospitals for over a hundred years. They are active against most bacteria, although not spores, and against viruses. Phenol (carbolic acid) used by Lord Lister to destroy bacteria in wounds and to prevent their access to wounds (*Lancet* 1867), was used as the standard disinfectant against which the efficiency and activity of others was measured in the Rideal-Walker test (1903). It is not now used for wounds since it is toxic and irritant and may cause local tissue damage and remote kidney damage.

Modern clear-soluble phenolic compounds, e.g. *Hycolin, Clearsol, Stericol* and *Sudol* are more efficient than phenol and have fewer disadvantages, although *Sudol* is too corrosive for many uses.

The 'white fluids', including *Izal* and *White Cyllin* are derived from coal tar. They are effective, relatively cheap and suitable for floor and surface disinfection and for decontamination of infected linen.

Chloroxylenols, e.g. Dettol are so easily inactivated by hard water and organic materials that they are of doubtful value.

Hexachlorophane is a chlorinated phenolic bacteriostatic agent which was widely used combined with a compatible soap for skin cleansing, in particular hand-washing, in operating theatres and clinical areas. It is cumulative in action and is therefore most effective when used consistently and frequently. It is slow acting and particularly inhibits the growth of Gram-positive bacteria. In the early 1970s warnings were published concerning the possibility of toxic effects from absorption of hexachlorophane. Young babies are considered to be at greatest risk since they could be exposed to considerable amounts of the agent over the course of weeks of 'topping and tailing' and bathing. The use of hexachlorophane is now restricted to short-term use in some special hospital units.

Diguanides. Chlorhexidine (Hibitane) is a complex synthetic organic compound of the diguanide group, active against a wide range of bacteria particularly the Gram-positive organisms, less so against Gram-negative bacilli. Chlorhexidine in alcohol is an efficient, non-irritant skin germicide, and in aqueous solution is used for wound toilet and irrigation. Aqueous solutions are liable to contamination by Gram-negative organisms such as *Pseudomonas* sp.

A 4% chlorhexidine detergent solution (Hibiscrub) is an effective skin cleansing agent which is widely used for hand-washing and preoperative skin preparation.

A 4% chlorhexidine solution in isopropyl alcohol (Hibisol) may be used as an alternative to hand washing between patients in, for example, a surgical ward where a number of clean dressings are being performed in a short time. The hands are 'washed' with a small amount of the solution until dry and no other action, washing or drying, is necessary. This procedure does not replace the necessity for adequate washing and cleansing of the hands if they become soiled or after handling a dirty infected wound.

Quaternary ammonium compounds. These compounds, e.g. Roccal, Ziphiran, Cetavlon, have very good detergent properties but are selective in action, being of limited use against Gram-negative bacteria and having no effect on tubercle bacilli, while proving effective against Gram-positive organisms such as staphylococci. The compounds include cationic, anionic and non-ionic solutions; if a cationic and an anionic solution are mixed the bacteriostatic activity of both is neutralized. They are also neutralized by soaps, hard water and various chemicals and have a peculiar adsorptive property. If the practice of moistening cotton wool balls by direct contact with the mouth of a bottle containing a quaternary ammonium is permitted, the solution in the bottle becomes progressively more inactive until only coloured water remains because the active agent is adsorbed on to the succession of wool balls. Not only will the remaining fluid be inactive but it will almost certainly become bacterially contaminated and cause infection when used for subsequent aseptic procedures. They cannot therefore be recommended for use.

QAC/Diguanide mixtures. E.g. Savlon (chlorhexidine and cetrimide) overcome some of the disadvantages of QACs, for use as skin disinfectants only. To avoid contamination risks it should be produced for use in small quantities, autoclaved at in-use concentration. It is therefore too expensive for any other disinfectant procedures.

Alcohols. Isopropyl alcohol 70% is an effective skin germicide. Greater concentrations are less effective since water is essential to the transfer of the antiseptic across the bacterial cell wall. It is also of use for disinfection of smooth surfaces. Chlorhexidine or iodine may be combined with alcohol for skin disinfection also.

Aldehydes. Glutaraldehyde is an effective disinfectant, non-volatile, but it may cause some irritation. It is effective against both Gram-positive and Gram-negative bacteria, including tubercle bacilli, and is supposedly sporicidal. It is most active in an alkaline solution but since it is unstable in this form, the alkali has to be added to the glutaraldehyde shortly before use; e.g. Cidex 25%, an aqueous solution of glutaraldehyde, is diluted to 2% with an alkali, 0.3% $NaCO_2$, and can be used for the chemical sterilization of articles which will not withstand heat processing, e.g. endoscopes (see page 85). (Formaldehyde 5% is an active, efficient disinfectant but has the disadvantage of a pungent smell and is very irritant to the skin, eyes and mucous membranes. Its only use now is for terminal disinfection of premises following smallpox infection.)

The following table gives examples of most situations where a disinfectant or antiseptic is appropriate, and indicates appropriate agents. Solutions should always be used in the strengths and dilutions recommended by the manufacturers. This list is not intended to be fully comprehensive. Excellent examples of suggested specific disinfec-

Disinfectant Guidelines

Site	Group	Example
Skin Hands	Diguanide	Chlorhexidine detergent solution, e.g. Hibiscrub, Hibisol
	Iodophors (Halogen)	Betadine, Disadine, Wescodyne
Preoperative preparation	Diguanide	Chlorhexidine in spirit—Hibitane detergent solution—Hibiscrub
	Alcohol	Isopropyl alcohol 70%
	Iodophors	Betadine, Disadine, etc.
Cleansing	QAC and Diguanide	Chlorhexidine and cetrimide, e.g. Savlon
Heat-sensitive instruments	Aldehyde	Glutaraldehyde, e.g. Cidex
Inanimate objects and surfaces	Phenolics (clear-soluble)	Hycolin, Clearsol
Special areas, e.g. SCBU, ITU	Halogen	Electrolytic sodium hypochlorite, e.g. Milton

tant guidelines for dealing with most situations and equipment can be found in Lowbury *et al.* (1982) and Maurer (1979), see Selected Further Reading.

Other anti-microbial preparations

Heavy metals. Silver nitrate and silver sulphadiazine are currently widely used in the treatment of burns. A practical disadvantage is the indelible black staining of bed and personal linen.

Oxidizing Agents. *Hydrogen peroxide* is an antiseptic which liberates oxygen when in contact with organic material. The effervescence helps mechanically to loosen slough and pus in a wound but any remaining fluid will be plain water with no antiseptic property.

Nebulized hydrogen peroxide 10 vol. has been found to be a suitable means of decontaminating intermittent positive pressure ventilators (Whitby 1968).

COLD

Freezing as a method of killing micro-organisms is not satisfactory for ordinary use because the survival rate of organisms in low temperatures varies considerably. Refrigeration is, however, an excellent method for preserving food, sera, etc., when the temperature is kept at about 4°C. Organisms are not killed by this method but they do not multiply. Perishable goods should be placed in the refrigerator immediately. If they are allowed to stay in a warm atmosphere for several hours organisms present in them will have a chance of multiplying and refrigeration after this time will be useless. Preformed toxins are not destroyed by refrigeration and no amount of cooling after they have been formed will make the food safe to eat.

DRYING

Many organisms are killed by drying and this factor limits the natural spread of many diseases. Spores, however, can withstand remaining dry for many months or even years and, as a practical method of killing bacteria, drying is unsatisfactory.

ULTRA-VIOLET LIGHT

Prolonged exposure to fresh air and sunlight is perhaps the oldest and most pleasant anti-infection measure. Ultra-violet rays reduce the number of air-borne bacteria but the practical value of an ultra-violet light installation as a means of killing bacteria in a hospital is minimal and its efficiency limited by disadvantageous physical properties.

1. Light travels in straight lines and does not penetrate. Only the surface of an object in direct line with the ultra-violet source is irradiated, any bacteria in 'the shadows' are totally unaffected.

2. Direct exposure to ultra-violet light causes conjunctival damage, so that either dark glasses must be worn or the light source screened.

3. Bacterial kill is not instantaneous. Neither human beings nor air passing at normal speed through a doorway with an overhead source will receive adequate exposure.

8 Diagnostic Microbiology

Laboratory tests are prescribed by the clinician in charge of a patient for various reasons. For example, the test may be to find out which particular organism is causing an obvious infection, or it may be to confirm or to eliminate a specific site or system as the focus of infection. The patient may apparently have recovered from an infection and the test prescribed is to check that he is free from the causative organism, or a specimen may be one of a series sent at regular intervals to monitor progress.

The clinician may consult with the microbiologist about the suitability of certain tests, for expert interpretation of laboratory findings or for advice on antibiotic therapy; he frequently delegates to the nursing staff the responsibility for obtaining appropriate specimens.

The laboratory staff can only examine the material and information presented to them, and the diagnosis, management, or treatment of patients may depend on the results which they report back to the clinician. Collecting specimens at the correct time, using the correct technique and despatching them without delay to the designated laboratory is therefore of critical importance. If the material presented to the laboratory is of poor quality then the result of the test reported back to the clinician will be unreliable.

COLLECTION OF SPECIMENS FOR BACTERIOLOGICAL EXAMINATION

The objectives are:

1. To collect an adequate amount of tissue or fluid uncontaminated by organisms from any outside source, but preserving any organisms which may present.

2. To ensure that the specimen is correctly identified by labelling, and sent to the laboratory with an accurately completed request form.

3. To transport the specimen from the patient to the laboratory safely and with the minimum of delay.

As a general rule the more material sent for examination, the greater the chance of isolating a causative organism. For example, it is preferable to send a few millilitres of pus aspirated with a sterile syringe and needle than to send a swab dipped in the pus.

Specimens are readily contaminated by poor techniques such as allowing urine to flow over the vulva before collecting it in the container, or by the use of unsterile equipment. Specimens should be collected in sterile laboratory containers, with the exception of faeces (clean container) and sputum (clean container free from respiratory organisms).

Ideally, samples should be collected before the commencement of antibiotic therapy. When it is necessary to test during a course of antibiotic treatment, the specimen should be collected just before a dose is given.

Similarly when an antiseptic is used for cleaning or packing a wound or body cavity, a specimen should be collected at the commencement of the dressing procedure to minimize the risk of also collecting antiseptic. The presence of antibiotic or antiseptic in the specimen container may destroy organisms which are in fact active in the patient and this will affect laboratory tests. Such treatment should be noted on the request form accompanying the specimen.

It is important to ensure that every specimen is clearly identified by a label giving the name and location of the patient and the date. The accompanying request form should give any relevant data, e.g. a provisional diagnosis, pyrexia, wound infection, chemotherapy, as well as the patient's name, age, sex and location; it must be legible.

Culture plates, used in the ward for direct plating of eye swabs, should always be labelled with wax pencil, on the base and not the lid. This prevents errors if the lids are inadvertently exchanged during transit or processing. Plates are stored base uppermost for ease of handling.

The sooner specimens reach the laboratory the greater the chance of any organisms present surviving and being identified. With the exception of blood culture samples, which should be placed in a 37°C incubator, immediately if possible, specimens which cannot be sent to the laboratory within a short time should be placed in a specimen refrigerator at 4°C. Some laboratories issue containers of sterile *transport medium* into which the tip of the swab stick is inserted. The purpose of transport medium is to preserve the organisms in the same condition and numbers as when present in the patient. It is effective for about 24 hours and should not be refrigerated or incubated.

Any specimen may contain pathogens. To avoid spreading organisms to other people or to the environment it is most important to avoid contamination of the outside of specimen containers and to ensure that they are securely closed and carefully handled. In the event of an *accidental spill* pour a small quantity of standard hospital disinfectant (e.g. Hycolin or domestic bleach) on to the spilt material. Wearing a pair of disposable gloves and using paper towel or newspaper, mop up the spill. Contain the paper, debris and gloves within a waterproof bag for safe disposal. Wash the hands thoroughly.

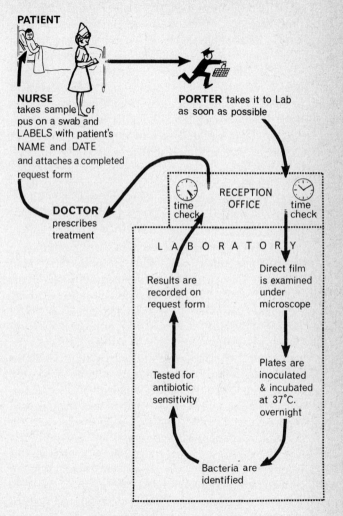

Fig. 20. The sequence of laboratory identification of bacteria from infected material.

If a specimen container leaks, not only are the porter and the laboratory staff at risk from accidental infection, but, since other contaminating bacteria can get into such a container even more easily than the specimen can leak out, a false answer to the test may be reported.

Delay *en route* to the laboratory is another factor which may affect the bacteria collected from a patient, particularly if the specimens are left in a warm place. For instance, a swab taken from a wound may dry out, causing the death of sensitive organisms, and this will result in a false negative report. Conversely, organisms multiply very fast in warm urine, so that the laboratory count of bacteria in a delayed specimen could be out of all proportion to that of the original specimen and a false positive report issued.

Nose and throat swabs. Swabs from the nose and throat are usually taken together, one swab for both tonsils and another for both nostrils; organisms causing sore throats are sometimes carried in the nose and failure to take nose swabs may mean that the organisms here are missed.

The patient is placed facing a strong source of light and the tongue is depressed. The swab should never be removed from its sterile tube until everything is ready for taking the specimen. When taking a throat swab care should be taken to avoid touching the mouth or tongue with the swab, which should be gently rubbed over the pillars of the fauces and any area with a lesion or visible exudate.

When taking nasal swabs it is important to ensure that the swab reaches as far back as possible on each side; this can usually be done by tilting the patient's head back and using a gentle twisting movement. With babies and very young children wooden swab sticks are often too large to get into the nostrils and many hospitals supply fine wire swabholders covered with a tiny wisp of cotton wool. Care is needed to avoid damage to the delicate mucous membranes with these swabs. Swabs should be replaced in the sterile containers immediately, to avoid contamination with airborne organisms.

The normal healthy nose is virtually dry, therefore when routine screening is carried out to check staphylococcal carriage the swab should be moistened with sterile distilled water. In this case nasal swabs should be taken from the anterior nares and the swab directed upwards in the tip of the nose and gently rotated to collect any secretion.

Ear swabs. The same type of swab stick is used for ear swabs as for nose and throat swabs, and care should be taken that no antibiotics or other chemotherapeutic or antiseptic material has been used in the ear within three hours of taking the swab.

Wound swabs. Wound swabs are usually taken when a dressing is being changed; the same type of swab stick is used as for ear, nose and throat swabs. The swab should be rotated to collect as much pus or exudate as possible. It is then immediately replaced in the container before any antiseptic or cleansing lotion is applied, immersed in transport medium.

Aspirations. Large quantities of material for microbiological investigation are usually taken by syringe and may be transferred directly from this syringe to a sterile bottle. Pleural, ascitic and synovial fluids are collected into a sterile bottle containing an anticoagulant; 20–30 ml is an adequate amount for bacterial examination unless tuberculosis is suspected when the whole aspirate should be sent to the laboratory. Cerebrospinal fluid should be collected in dry sterile containers. Fluids requiring a cell count should be put into two sterile bottles appropriately labelled; the second one should be used for the count, since the first aspirate may contain extraneous blood cells introduced into the needle as it went through the tissues.

Sputum. The sputum is never free from organisms since material originating in the bronchi and alveoli has to pass through the pharynx and mouth which always have a normal commensal population of bacteria. The specimen containers need to be clean but not sterile; they must however be free from organisms of respiratory origin and most laboratories now use waxed paper or plastic disposable containers with secure lids. Disinfectant must not be put in sputum pots which are to be sent for microbiological investigation.

Care should be taken that the material sent for investigation is in fact sputum and not saliva. Patients who have difficulty in bringing up phlegm should be encouraged to cough first thing in the morning. Patients with coughs usually have mucopurulent, or purulent flecks in the specimen. The specimen should be as large as possible and it is better to wait until an adequate specimen can be produced than to waste laboratory time on minute specimens of saliva. When the specimen has been coughed up the bacterial population alters in proportion rapidly; it is therefore important that the specimen should be sent to the laboratory immediately.

Specimens of sputum in cases of suspected tuberculosis. The tubercle bacillus, *Mycobacterium tuberculosis*, may sometimes be thinly distributed in the sputum and a large quantity of material must therefore be submitted for examination on direct film and for cultures to be made. The bacillus is most likely to be present in the purulent flecks. It is usual to send three specimens of sputum taken on different days when looking for the tubercle bacillus; the results may not be available for six weeks or even longer, because cultures grow slowly. Patients with suspected pulmonary tuberculosis who are not producing any sputum usually have the stomach contents aspirated on three successive mornings before any food or liquid is taken. The total aspirate is sent to the laboratory as soon as possible.

Urine. Specimens of urine should normally be taken in the early morning when the urine has accumulated in the bladder over night: all specimens from one patient are then roughly comparable. If they are taken at other times the urine may sometimes be diluted due to a high fluid intake. Early morning specimens are not, of course, possible in out-patient clinics, but they should be the rule for in-patients. In examination for tubercle bacilli in the urine, where the organisms are likely to be very scanty, the whole of the specimen should be sent in a sterile bottle.

Specimens of urine from male patients should be 'mid-stream specimens'; that is to say, after the skin surrounding the urethral meatus has been cleansed the patient micturates and the middle portion of the stream is collected directly into a sterile container to avoid contamination of the specimen with organisms normally present on the skin.

The collection of an uncontaminated mid-stream specimen from a female patient is not easy and should be carried out under nursing supervision when possible. The external genitalia and then the urethral meatus should be carefully cleansed. The patient micturates with the labia separated, and the middle portion of the stream is collected directly into a wide-mouthed sterile container.

A urine specimen from a patient who has an indwelling catheter should be aspirated, with a sterile syringe and needle, through the catheter wall. If the catheter has no aspiration insert and is too rigid for safe puncture, the drainage tubing insert may be used. It is much less satisfactory to collect the specimen from the end of the catheter. The sample should never be taken from the drainage bag.

Urine specimens should reach the laboratory within 1 hr or be refrigerated at 4°C until transported so that the numbers and types of different bacteria can be accurately assessed.

Faeces. Specimens of stools for examination should be sent in clean but unsterile containers which may be sub-

sequently burnt. Some bacteriologists allow rectal swabs
for the detection of the organisms causing food poisoning
or dysentery. These swabs are of the same type as those
used for wounds and the nose and throat, and care should
be taken to pass the swab through the anus right into the
rectum. Such swabs, to be satisfactory, should show clear
evidence of faecal contamination in any case. It is advisable
to send a specimen of stool as well if this is available so that
the amount of pus, blood and mucus and the consistency of
the specimen can be estimated.

Specimens of stools for parasites. Segments of *tapeworm*
can be seen with ease in any specimen of stool and the
worm will continue to grow and shed segments unless the
head is dislodged; it is therefore important to search for this
in every specimen passed by the patient after treatment.
Stool specimens should be strained through fine black
material under a running tap, the tapeworm segments will
be retained and can be sent to the laboratory for identification of the species and for confirmation of the presence
of the head.

Many intestinal worms shed their *ova* into the faeces;
they can only be seen microscopically and a fresh specimen
of stool should be sent to the laboratory in a suitable
container. Threadworms lay their ova on the perianal skin;
swabs of this area should therefore be taken as the ova will
not be seen in stool specimens. The sticky side of trans-
parent Sellotape is used for this purpose and is pressed on
to the skin of the perianal area, in the early morning and
before defaecation. The Sellotape should then be placed
adhesive side down on to a glass slide which is sent to the
laboratory.

Specimens of stool for amoebae. The parasites of amoebic
dysentery, *Entamoeba histolytica,* exist in a free-living
motile form and in the form of non-motile cysts. Both

forms are characteristic in their fresh state and a diagnosis of amoebic dysentery can be made from a fresh specimen of stool. The free-living form, however, becomes non-motile very easily in older specimens when the temperature has fallen, and both forms are more difficult to recognize when they are dead. It is therefore essential that specimens of stool for amoebae should be sent to the laboratory as soon as they are passed and should be examined immediately. It may be necessary to examine many specimens before the amoebae are seen.

Eye swabs. Either a bacteriologist's wire loop or a fine cotton wool swab should be used. Rub gently over the conjunctiva in the lower conjunctival sac, taking care to hold the swab parallel to the cornea and to avoid contamination by touching the lids. Conjunctival swabs should be inoculated on to an agar plate at the bedside as the lysozyme normally present in tears is antibacterial in action.

Purulent conjunctivitis in babies may be due to the gonococcus, which is a very delicate organism and may be killed if the swabs are allowed to dry or get cold. In some hospitals it is a routine procedure in cases of purulent conjunctivitis to take two swabs. One of these swabs is placed in transport medium, the other swab is not, so that direct films of the pus can be stained and examined in the laboratory.

Vaginal swabs. The specimens should be taken from as high in the vaginal vault as possible after introduction of a speculum to separate the walls. If *Trichomonas* infection is suspected the swab should be broken off in Fineberg's medium. Other cervical, urethral and vaginal swabs should be broken off in Stuart's transport medium. Specimens may also be taken with a teated pipette contained in a test tube.

Blood cultures. Samples of blood are usually taken by the medical staff and are used for direct isolation of pathogenic organisms in cases of septicaemia or other blood-borne infection. The specimens should be taken with full aseptic precautions; a dry, sterile syringe is used and a fresh sterile needle replaces that used for the venepuncture to inoculate the bottle of culture medium.

Success or failure in isolating organisms present in the blood stream is largely dependent upon taking the specimen at the right time and putting it into suitable medium for cultivation, and in this the nursing staff can give valuable assistance.

The clinician will tell the microbiologist what organism he thinks may be present; the microbiologist will choose the correct medium; and the blood is put directly into one of more bottles of this fluid. Organisms are most likely to be present in the blood stream in the greatest number when the temperature is at its highest, so that the most favourable time for taking a blood culture is at the peak of the temperature. The ward sister's knowledge of the patient's previous temperature range will help in predicting when this is likely to be, and it is her duty to keep a watch on his temperature and inform the medical officer or the laboratory when this is rising. With all requests for blood cultures certain information should be sent to the laboratory:

1. The time the blood culture was taken and the patient's temperature at that time.
2. The length of time the patient has been ill.
3. Any inflammatory lesions the patient may have, e.g. pneumonia, septic wound, urinary infection and the microbiology of these lesions if known.
4. Any chemotherapeutic treatment the patient may be having, and when he had his last dose. (Chemotherapeutic drugs for this purpose would include antibiotics.)

Serum for detection of antibodies. For this investigation 10 ml of blood should be taken into a dry tube or bottle containing no anticoagulant, and allowed to clot.

Specific antibodies do not appear in the serum for several days. It is the usual procedure to take blood at the beginning of a disease and then again after 10 days; the specimens are examined together in the laboratory. An increase in the amount of antibodies in the second specimen will be an indication of continued stimulation by the organism which must therefore be present in the patient. By comparing two specimens more information is gained, although single samples are sometimes helpful.

It is important that samples are accompanied by full details of:

1. The clinical history.
2. The length of time the patient has been ill.
3. Any history of a previous attack of the disease, with dates.
4. Any history of immunization

COLLECTION OF MATERIAL FOR DIAGNOSIS OF FUNGAL INFECTIONS

Hair. Samples of broken and infected hairs should be removed with forceps and sent to the laboratory in a clean sealed envelope or suitably dry specimen container so that the base of the hair can be examined and cultured. Some fungi fluoresce in ultra-violet light and a lamp may be used to identify infected hairs.

Nails. The whole thickness of the nail or deep scrapings should be sent in a dry container to the laboratory.

Skin lesions. The skin should be cleaned with alcohol. Epidermal scales scraped from the active edge of a lesion or the roof of any vesicles should be sent to the laboratory in a dry container.

Other specimens. Sputum, ear swabs, body fluids and curettings are collected in the same way as specimens for bacteriological examination.

COLLECTION OF SPECIMENS FOR VIROLOGICAL INVESTIGATION

Virus laboratories usually supply special transport media and should be consulted before specimens are taken. In addition to the patient data sent with a specimen for bacteriological examination (page 101) the virologist will require the date of the onset of the illness, and the patient's immunization record particularly of any inoculation within one month.

If the specimen cannot be delivered to the laboratory within 1 hr of collection it should be refrigerated at 4°C.

When viral disease is suspected several different specimens may be taken.

Central nervous system disease: Cerebrospinal fluid, brain, blood, faeces, throat swabs or washings.

Respiratory disease: Sputum, throat swabs or washings.

Eye disease: Conjunctival swabs or scrapings.

Skin lesions: Vesicle or pustule fluid in capillary tubes, air-dried slides from scrapings of macules or papules.

Serological tests are often undertaken and for these 5–10 ml of clotted blood are required. Two blood samples may be needed, the first taken as soon as possible after the onset of illness, the second 2–3 weeks later so that antibody levels (titres) can be compared. Alternatively, diagnosis may be based on the demonstration of specific IgM antibody in a single, early blood sample.

ISOLATION OF THE CAUSATIVE
ORGANISM FROM INFECTED MATERIAL

The microbiologist identifies an organism in material which is sent to him by a number of tests which have been designed to tell him a series of facts:

1. Morphology (i.e. size and shape) of the organism and its staining properties
2. Conditions for growth
3. Cultural characteristics
4. Biochemical tests
5. Resistance
6. Serological tests
7. Pathogenicity tests in experimental animals

Morphology of the organism
The organisms present in any specimen sent to the microbiologist are examined to determine their size, shape and other specific characteristics. They may be from 0.3 μm to 14 μm in length (μm = 0.001 mm). They may be round, rod-shaped or spiral. They may grow in pairs, clusters or chains, and a given culture may contain organisms of irregular size and shape. They may possess flagella or may bear spores. To make them readily visible they are stained with various dyes in different ways to distinguish them according to the effects of various staining processes.

Staining. The bacterial kingdom can be roughly divided into two by the action of a staining technique called *Gram's method,* which consists of staining the cells with a basic dye, methyl violet, and afterwards treating with iodine. The film stain is then decolorized with alcohol or acetone, until no more is removed. The organisms are subsequently counterstained with a red contrasting coloured dye, e.g. safranin. Gram-positive organisms are those which retain the methyl violet and appear purple under the microscope. Gram-negative ones are those which do not retain the dye and are stained red by the counterstain. Hence bacteria are divided into Gram-positive and Gram-negative groups and this grouping, together with the baterial shape, cocci, bacilli or very short ovoid organisms called coccobacilli, gives the bacteriologist a start in his identification.

The tubercle bacillus (*Mycobacterium tuberculosis*) and some related organisms are stained only with difficulty by Gram's stain, but can be reliably stained by using hot, strong carbol fuchsin, which is impossible to remove from them with acid and alcohol. This is the basis of the *Ziehl-Neelsen* stain and the organisms so stained are said to be 'acid-alcohol fast'.

Organisms which are able to move by means of flagella or hair-like structures which may be placed in various positions on the bacterial body can be stained by special techniques only. Spirochaetes such as *Treponema pallidum,* the organism responsible for syphilis, are capable of movement by bending their spiral bodies and the rate and character of the movement is characteristic. Some organisms such as the pneumococcus are surrounded by a clear capsule which can be demonstrated by special stains.

Conditions of growth

It is the usual procedure, when endeavouring to isolate an organism, to put infected material into a sterile mixture containing nutriments which are suitable to encourage the growth of likely organisms. Such mixtures of foodstuffs are called 'culture media' and many have a meat infusion, like clear soup, as a basis. These liquids are stored in sterile bottles; a swab previously dipped in infected material is broken into one of these and if bacteria are present they will multiply on incubation and the bacterial growth will show as an opacity in the fluid. The meat infusion may be mixed with hot melted agar-agar, poured into flat dishes called Petri dishes or into screw-capped bottles, set aslant, and allowed to set. Infected material is spread on the surface of these using a fine wire loop.

To encourage the growth of various organisms certain other substances can be added to the basic medium either to enrich it, or to make it selective. For example, amino acids, proteins in the form of serum, plasma or whole blood, or vitamins may be used as enrichments.

Selective media are those which contain substances known to inhibit certain organisms or groups of organisms. They are also useful in the detection of pathogenic organisms from material such as stools and throat swabs, both of which are normally full of organisms. If unselective enriched media are used, the normal non-pathogenic organisms may overgrow the sparse pathogens and make their detection difficult. In practice there are selective media for many species and certain media have become routine for primary inoculation of material from most sites.

Cultural characteristics

In order to ascertain the cultural characteristic of an organism, infected material is introduced into suitable fluid and solid media. On the latter it is spread thinly over the whole plate with a wire loop, which is sterilized in a flame before and after use. The inoculated media are then put into incubators adjusted to a constant temperature. In medical microbiology 37°C is the temperature of primary incubation, because the majority of human pathogens have this as their optimum temperature.

Many organisms, such as the staphylococcus or the diphtheria bacillus, grow best in an atmosphere containing oxygen; they grow well therefore in air and are said to be aerobic organisms. Some, such as the gonococcus, the organism causing gonorrhoea, grow best in an atmosphere containing carbon dioxide, and for isolation of this

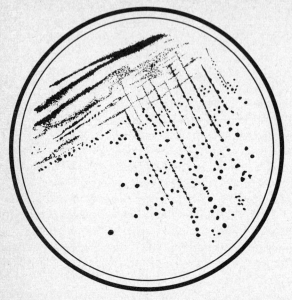

Fig. 21. Colonies on a plate spread by the method of parallel streaks. A small portion of the material to be examined is spread over the surface by successive parallel strokes of a wire loop.

organism from an infected patient the inoculated plates are put into a tin which contains 5% carbon dioxide and the tin is put in the incubator. Other organisms, such as *Clostridium tetani,* cannot grow where there is free oxygen, and to grow these organisms conditions must be made anaerobic by placing the plates in a tin or jar, partially evacuating the air which is then replaced with hydrogen. The hydrogen is combined with the residual oxygen to produce completely anaerobic conditions. These are strictly anaerobic organisms, but there are some facultative anaerobes, that is to say they are equipped with enzymes which allow them to utilize either aerobic or anaerobic respiration.

It is usual to leave the plates undisturbed in the incubator overnight (18–24 h.) before looking for growth. Some organisms grow slowly and often no growth is visible to the naked eye at this time. With other organisms, along the lines of inoculation there will be heaped colonies of growing organisms, ranging from 0.1 mm to 4 mm in diameter. These colonies, each containing many organisms, all of the same kind, have developed by division o the initial ones put on with the loop. Their size, shape, colour, consistency and effect on the surrounding medium are all of importance and characteristic of the species. Instead of isolated colonies the organisms may have spread in a film all over the plate; organisms which do this are those which are highly motile, that is capable of movement in the thin film of water which covers the surface of the plate.

Biochemical tests

Certain biochemical tests have been found useful to differentiate various bacteria. The majority of these tests are designed to detect the presence of enzymes in the organisms which bring about a specific chemical reaction. The *Shigella* group of organisms, those causing dysentery, are morphologically and culturally identical, but can be differentiated by the different carbohydrates which they can break down by enzyme action, so as to use them as a source of energy. If these organisms are grown in medium containing mannitol as a source of carbohydrate, certain of them can break this down, and the breakdown products will be acid in reaction. If, therefore, an indicator is added which will show acid production by its change in colour, this change indicates the ability to ferment mannitol and tells the bacteriologist that this organism may be *Shigella sonnei,* or one of the *Shigella flexneri* organisms, if other reactions also fit in with what is known of these organisms.

Some organisms are soluble in bile; a *Pneumococcus* may be differentiated from a viridans type of *Streptococcus* by tests making use of this principle.

The ability to break down and use starch is a characteristic which differentiates the one strain of diphtheria bacillus from the other members of the genus *Corynebacterium,* and is a useful differentiating test. The ability to form indole in a medium containing tryptophan is a characteristic of many non-pathogenic Gram-negative intestinal organisms. There are many other examples used diagnostically, all reflecting fundamental metabolic processes which have by experience been found useful in differentiating one organism from another.

A relatively recent development of importance has been the production of miniaturized kits made of disposable plastic which contain materials for performing standard biochemical tests that are often used for the routine identification of organisms of medical interest. One such is the French API system, supplying a large number of tests (often 20 or more) in a small space and using very small amounts of reagents; it allows rapid accurate bacterial identification even in laboratories with limited facilities.

Resistance

The resistance of an organism to temperature, drying, acid, antiseptics, dyes, chemotherapeutic agents and antibodies, is a help in diagnosis as well as a help in treatment and prevention of spread. As we have already seen, those organisms which have not the power of forming spores are relatively less resistant to heat than the spore-bearing organisms. Some haemolytic streptococci will be killed if kept at 60°C for 30 minutes; certain other streptococci, may be differentiated by a heat resistance test, since they withstand 60°C for 30 minutes. Very heat resistant spores of certain organisms such as *Bacillus anthracis* will withstand 100°C for a considerable time.

The sensitivity of various organisms to antibiotics, although it may be of value in differentiating strains, is of more value as a guide to therapy.

Serology

An organism isolated from infected material contains numerous antigens; if these are mixed with serum containing known specific antibodies prepared by injection of a known organism into an experimental animal, and the unknown organism reacts with the specific antiserum, the antigens in the unknown organism must be the same as or closely related to those which were used to immunize the experimental animal. Antigen–antibody reactions are used a great deal in bacteriology, the union of antigen with antibody often being associated with an altered physical state of the mixture such as a clumping of bacterial cells, which enables it to be seen. Use is also made of such reactions, as we have seen before, in detecting unknown antibodies in the patient's serum, the serum being mixed with known organisms acting as antigens. This principle forms the basis of the Widal test for enteric fever (Fig. 22).

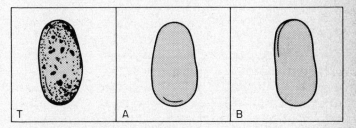

Fig. 22. Slide agglutination seen by naked eye. A culture of bacteria from a suspected typhoid carrier has been mixed with drops of antisera prepared against *Salmonella typhi* (T), *Salm. paratyphi* (A), and *Salm. paratyphi* (B). It has been agglutinated by T but not by A or B. Therefore the organism is identified as the typhoid bacillus.

Inoculation of infected material into laboratory animals

Some infectious agents cannot be cultured on artificial media, and their presence can only be detected by producing the disease in an experimental animal which is

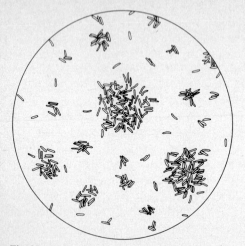

Fig. 23. Agglutination as seen under the microscope.

known to be susceptible. Tissues from the animal may show changes typical of the disease. For example, when tubercle bacilli cannot be found in the urine, tuberculosis may sometimes be produced in a guinea-pig by injection with some of the infected fluid.

These are the means then, by which the bacteriologist is able to identify organisms present in the material which is sent to him, but it will be obvious that this identification is bound to take time. In rare cases the organisms can be seen in direct films of the material and their appearance will be diagnostic. More commonly 18 hr are necessary for the organisms to be grown on media and only then can the various differential tests be applied.

In specimens taken from sites which are normally inhabited by organisms, such as the respiratory tract, the bowel and lesions involving the skin, the bacterial flora will be mixed and before identification can begin the organisms must be separated and isolated in pure culture.

DEMONSTRATION OF ANTIBODIES IN PATIENT'S SERUM

The diagnosis of infectious disease by demonstrating the presence of antibodies in the patient's serum is discussed under Immunity in Chapter 5; it is as well to note that the inference to be drawn from the presence of specific antibodies in a patient's serum is limited. All that can be deduced is that the patient has at some time been subjected to the specific antigen under test. A present attack of the disease is best diagnosed by taking repeated samples of serum and showing that these contain an increase in antibody content or 'titre'.

HYPERSENSITIVITY TESTS SUGGESTING A PREVIOUS DOSE OF A PATHOGENIC ORGANISM

Hypersensitivity reactions may be: *(a)* Immediate, when they are an allergic response of the body to certain foreign proteins and occur in the cellular structures affected, e.g. hay fever. *(b)* Delayed, when the response is dependent on immunologically activated lymphocytes reaching the site of entry of the antigen. The delay is due to the fact that the lymphocytes have to migrate to this site, e.g. tuberculin test.

This reaction of sensitivity is the basis of the tuberculin test. A positive reaction does not necessarily mean that the patient has the active disease at the time of the test, but that he has at some previous date had a dose of the antigen. The diagnostic value of a positive tuberculin test is therefore limited. Many people have a primary dose of tuberculosis in their childhood or adolescence, which they overcome without difficulty and with no clinical symptoms, and the majority of adults are therefore tuberculin positive.

NON-SPECIFIC TESTS

There are certain tests which have been found by experience to be positive in certain diseases, although the reasons are unknown. The tests are mainly antigen–antibody reactions. The patient's serum in certain diseases contains an antibody which reacts with an antigen which did not stimulate its production, that is to say, one other than the infecting agent. It is probable that this infecting agent and the test antigen are, however, chemically and antigenically related. This happens in some circumstances with the *Salmonella* group of diseases.

Weil-Felix reaction

An attack of typhus stimulates the production of antibodies which react with a certain strain of *Proteus,* and in this test the *Proteus* organism is used as the antigen. More specific tests, using the typhus *Rickettsia* itself, are replacing this test.

Cold agglutinins

The infective agent or agents responsible for virus pneumonia have never been isolated, so that specific antigen–antibody reactions are not possible. It has been shown, however, that certain patients with this disease develop in their serum antibodies which agglutinate human group O red blood cells at a low temperature. This is of some help in diagnosis.

There are many examples, too numerous to mention, of non-specific serological tests used in diagnosis of past or present infectious diseases, and as more is known of the antigenic and chemical nature of the infective agents, the reasons for the phenomena may become apparent.

THE LABORATORY REPORT

Features described in the report

Macroscopy. The gross appearance of the specimen received by the laboratory may be important information to the clinician assessing the report, e.g. *Staphylococcus aureus* present in saliva may be due to nasal carriage of the organism, but the same organism in a true specimen of sputum is most likely to be due to severe chest infection.

Microscopy. Information is gained from looking at prepared slides under the microscope, such as the presence of cells, casts or crystals, yeasts or fungi, parasites or their ova. It is usual, when tuberculosis is suspected, for the reports to state 'ZN positive' or 'ZN negative' with 'further report to follow' because of the time required to obtain a definitive answer on culture. A negative Ziehl-Neelsen test does not mean that the patient is not tuberculous. It means that tubercle bacilli were not seen in the part of the single specimen examined. A positive report usually means that there were large numbers of tubercle bacilli present, i.e. the patient has active disease.

Culture. This is the information gained from culturing the organism and its identification.

1. The organism is named, e.g. *Streptococcus* (the family name). This may be followed by the abbreviation sp(p). = species, or a further identification of the member of the family, e.g. *Streptococcus faecalis* or *Streptococcus pyogenes*.

2. The growth of the organism may be described in terms of quality, e.g. heavy or moderate, or it may be described quantitively, e.g. the number of bacteria per litre of urine, expressed as $> 10^8$/litre.

3. The laboratory may report on the presence or absence of a particular organism only, because the clinician does not require any other information. This is described as a screening test and the report states, for example 'No *Salmonella* sp. isolated'.

Antibiotic sensitivity. The sensitivity of a pathogen to a range of antibiotics reported as a guide to the clinician if he consideres that the patient requires antibiotic therapy. s = sensitive, r = resistant.

Serology. The dosage of certain antibiotics, e.g. gentamicin, is controlled in some patients by the estimation of serum levels of the drug. Trough and peak levels are usually reported in μg/ml. Trough specimens are taken immediately before a dose of the drug is given and represent the lowest level reached by the drug. Peak levels conversely represent maximum drug levels and are taken soon after a dose of the drug has been administered and absorbed, often ½–1 hour after a dose.

Antibody titres may be reported in figures, e.g. 1 in 200, or may be interpreted by the microbiologists, e.g. 'shows a significant rise in titre' (a titre is the highest dilution at which antibody is detected).

The use of laboratory reports

Laboratory reports should only be interpreted with knowledge of the clinical condition of the patient. The fact that a pathogen and antibiotic sensitivities are reported does not necessarily imply that the patient must be given therapy; he may already be recovering from the infection. The fact that no organism was isolated does not necessarily mean that the site was sterile; it could be the result of poor technique in obtaining the specimen.

On the other hand, reports may contribute towards establishing a diagnosis, the prescription of treatment or further surgery, or they may be used in series as a measure of a patient's progress. Reports give information on which to base decisions concerning the nursing care of patients, the pattern of the day's work in a ward, the movement and grouping of patients and measures necessary to contain, or to prevent the spread of infection.

9 A Guide to Common Pathogenic Bacteria

The aim of this chapter is to present some outstanding facts about common organisms which the nurse may use for quick reference when she meets them in laboratory reports.

Most of the organisms have two or even three names, and in the pages that follow the present international name used by microbiologists is given first, followed by the common names used in Britain before the international nomenclature was adopted. Abbreviations which are readily understood by those without professional bacteriological experience have been used in preference to the short correct version. For example, *Salm*. is used instead of *S*. for *Salmonella* and *Esch*. for *E*. meaning *Escherichia*.

THE MAIN DIVISIONS OF MICRO—ORGANISMS

The population of the microbiological world can be grouped into six divisions:

1. Non-branching organisms stained by crystal violet+iodine (Gram-positive) (staining, see page 113).
2. Non-branching organisms not stained by crystal violet+iodine (Gram-negative).
3. Branching organisms, Gram-positive and Gram-negative.

4. Organisms stained by the Ziehl Neelsen technique (acid-fast).

5. Some spirochaetes which are often difficult to stain by the techniques mentioned above.

6. Organisms only seen inside stained cells (viruses and rickettsiae) or by means of an electron microscope.

1. GRAM-POSITIVE DIVISION

Streptococcus

Oval cocci in pairs or chains like strings of beads. Found everywhere. Many inhabit mucous membranes of man and animals, including mouth, upper respiratory tract and intestine. Many live in food, especially milk and dairy products, where they are found with the *Lactobacillus*. Some kinds discolour or destroy red blood cells and are called 'haemolytic streptococci'.

PATHOGENIC

β-haemolytic *Streptococcus*

Str. pneumoniae (pneumococcus) cause of **primary pneumonia, meningitis, peritonitis**

POTENTIALLY PATHOGENIC

Str. faecalis (Lancefield Group D)

Str. viridans may cause **sub-acute bacterial endocarditis**

Str. pyogenes (Group A) cause of **tonsillitis, scarlet fever, acute nephritis, acute rheumatic fever, puerperal fever, wound infection, erysipelas, cellulitis**

Lancefield groups B C G

HARMLESS TO MAN
Hundreds of strains

Grouping of streptococci

Beta-haemolytic streptococci are grouped by identification of specific chemical antigens into 14 Lancefield groups A–O. Groups A, C and G are usually responsible for human streptococcal infections. Group A is the most virulent and is responsible for the majority of these infections. During an outbreak of streptococcal infection it may be necessary to distinguish between two or more Group A strains. This is done by serological tests which subdivide Group A strains into about 40 different Griffith types.

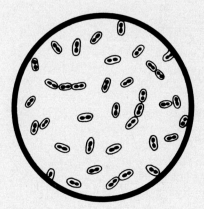

Fig. 24. *Streptococcus pneumoniae* stained to show capsules.

Staphylococcus

Spherical cocci in clusters like grapes. Found on mucous membranes, skin, and as a contaminant in air and soil.

PATHOGENIC	HARMLESS
Staphylococcus aureus, or coagulase-positive staphylococcus, sometimes called *Staph. pyogenes.* Usually enters through the skin, but may enter through mucous membranes. Spread by human carriers and found in about 50% of people, especially hospital staff. Cause of all kinds of **abscesses, boils, carbuncles, whitlows, styes, breast abscess, pemphigus neonatorum, infected wounds, pneumonia, and one form of food poisoning**	*Staphylococcus epidermis, Staphylococcus albus* and *Staphylococcus citreus.* Coagulase-negative, found in nose and on the skin, and in the environment

Typing of coagulase-positive staphylococci

Coagulase-positive staphylococci can be typed and identified by the effect of staphylococcal bacteriophage upon them. Bacteriophages are highly specific viruses not pathogenic to man, which attack and destroy susceptible bacteria. This typing is important to the infection control team; there are many types of *Staphylococcus* and the bacteriologist tries to find out which particular type is the cause of cross-infection in an outbreak. Swabs may be taken from staff and patients to identify the troublesome strain and to try to trace its spread from patient to patient. Sometimes the source may be the nose of an individual whose wound becomes infected, an example of bacteria which are saprophytic in one situation and pathogens in another. This is autoinfection.

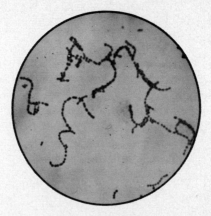

Fig. 25. Culture smear of *Streptococcus pyogenes* showing the characteristic chain arrangement of streptococci (× 1000).

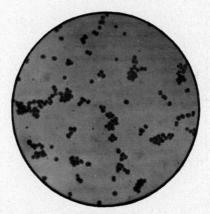

Fig. 26. Culture smear of *Staphyloccus aureus* showing characteristic clumping (× 1000).

Corynebacterium

Rod-shaped. Found on skin and mucous membranes particularly of the respiratory tract.

PATHOGENIC	HARMLESS
C. diphtheriae (diphtheria bacillus, or Klebs-Loeffler bacillus). Usual portal of entry is the upper respiratory tract, but occasionally the vagina, the skin or the conjunctiva. Spread by human carriers. Cause of **diphtheria**	*C. hofmannii, C. xerosis* and other diphtheroids, commonly found as skin commensals

C. diphtheriae is distinguished from the harmless members of the group by biochemical tests, but principally by exotoxin-production, which may be demonstrated by guinea pig inoculation. The Schick test is an intradermal test with toxin which determines a patient's susceptibility to diphtheria.

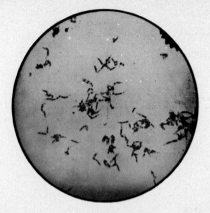

Fig. 27. Culture smear of *Corynebacterium diphtheriae* showing characteristic arrangement and uneven staining (× 1000).

Clostridium

Rods with spores which are wider than the parent organism, shaped like spindle, key or tennis racket. Found in the intestinal tract of man and animals and, of course, in soil. Anaerobe. Many members are harmless (*Clostridium sporogenes*) and even the pathogenic members may not cause disease unless the organisms or spores are carried into wounds, or tissues where conditions are exactly suitable for growth and toxin production.

PATHOGENIC

Cl. tetani, or *Bacillus tetani*. Produces exotoxin when carried into wounds. This poisons the anterior horn cell of the spinal cord thus affecting the motor nerves, producing an effect not unlike strychnine, resulting in the disease **tetanus**	*Cl. welchii (perfringens)* or *Bacillus welchii*. Produces toxin when carried into wounds involving muscle with damaged blood supply. The muscle infection produced is known as **gas gangrene.** Other important gas gangrene producers are *Cl. septique* and *Cl. oedematiens*	*Cl. botulinum*, or *Bacillus botulinum*. Produces toxin in tinned, potted or semi-cooked food, usually vegetable. The poisoned food when eaten causes acute toxaemia characterized by paralysis of the cranial motor nerves and of the diaphragm which is known as **botulism**

Certain strains of *Cl. perfringens* are associated with a mild form of food poisoning.

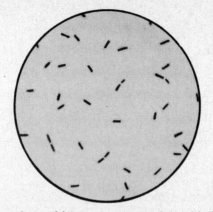

Fig. 28. *Clostridium welchii* showing characteristic brick-shaped bacilli (× 1000).

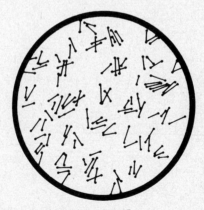

Fig. 29. Diagram showing delicate rod-shaped *Clostridium tetani*, with many round terminal spores, characteristically drum-shaped (× 1200).

Bacillus

Large rods with spores which do not swell the organisms. Spores very resistant to heat and other physical and chemical agents. Aerobe. Found in air, soil, water, dust, wool, hair, carcases.

PATHOGENIC	HARMLESS
B. anthracis, or anthrax bacillus. Enters through the skin, spores inhaled into the lungs or swallowed. Spread by animals and animal products, such as hides, hair, wool, infected carcases and bedding. Cause of **anthrax**	*B. subtilis.* Very widely distributed in dust
B. cereus is a cause of **toxic food poisoning** when ingested in large quantities. Otherwise non-pathogenic and widely distributed in the environment	

B. anthracis is distinguished from the harmless members of the group by biochemical tests and pathogenicity tests in animals.

B. cereus, an otherwise non-pathogenic organism, grows profusely in partly cooked rice and sometimes in other cereals from the spores that survive the cooking process. A toxin is elaborated that survives the final cooking and causes enteritis after ingestion.

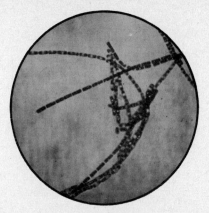

Fig. 30. Culture smear of *Bacillus anthracis* showing chain formation and many spores (× 900).

Candida

Candida albicans (Monilia) is an oval, yeast-like *fungus* which is strongly Gram-positive. In cultures and in tissues it frequently grows filamentous threads in addition to the usual budding yeast forms. It is found in the normal flora of mucous membranes in the mouth, intestinal tract and vagina. Occasionally, often in association with another pathological condition, immunological deficiency, or treatment with broad spectrum antibiotics, it becomes the dominant strain and infection results. Such infections are generally local, but very rarely they produce progressive systemic disease. This organism is resistant to all antibacterial antibiotics and flourishes in patients being so treated. Commonly transmitted from patient to patient in hospitals.

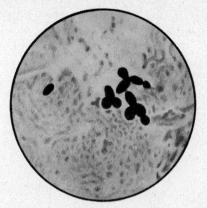

Fig. 31. Direct vaginal smear from a patient suffering from moniliasis. Note the characteristic dark staining, budding, yeast-like *Candida albicans* (× 1000).

2. GRAM-NEGATIVE DIVISION

Neisseria

Kidney-shaped bodies in pairs, often seen inside pus cells. Found on mucous membranes, particularly upper respiratory tract, genitourinary tract and conjunctiva.

PATHOGENIC		HARMLESS
N. gonorrhoeae, or gonococcus. Enters through mucous membrane of genitourinary tract or conjunctiva. Cause of **gonorrhoea** and some cases of **purulent ophthalmia.** Usually seen in direct smears of pus from urethritis and cervicitis	*N. meningitidis*, or meningococcus. Enters through mucous membrane of upper respiratory tract, thence to blood stream and central nervous system. Healthy nasopharyngeal carriers provide the reservoirs of infection. Cause of **cerebrospinal fever.** Also called **meningococcal meningitis.** Found in cerebrospinal fluid in cases of meningitis and usually easily seen in direct smears	*N. catarrhalis*, *N. pharyngeus*, commensals of the respiratory tract

Both these pathogenic organisms die very quickly outside the body and this must be remembered when material for culture is being taken.

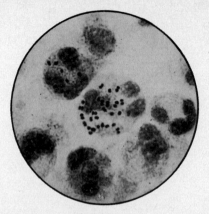

Fig. 32. Direct smear of urethral discharge from a patient suffering from acute gonorrhoea. Note characteristic intracellular *Neissaeria gonorrhoea* and close similarity to Fig. 33 (× 1000).

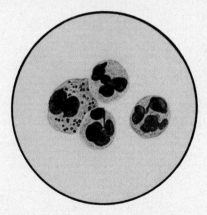

Fig. 33. Smear of cerebrospinal fluid from a case of *meningococcal* meningitis. Note pus cells with characteristic intracellular *Neisseria meningitidis* (× 475).

Haemophilus

Very small rod-shaped organisms, but varying greatly in length. Usually inhabit mucous membranes of man and animals.

PATHOGENIC   HARMLESS

Strains of *H. influenzae* found in the upper respiratory tract of older children and adults

H. ducreyi. Enters by mucous membrane of genital tract. Cause of **soft sore** or **soft chancre**

*H. influenzae,** or Pfeiffer's bacillus. Certain strains enter through upper respiratory tract and pass via blood stream into central nervous system. May also infect the conjunctiva. Cause of **meningitis** and **conjunctivitis.** Often found in patients with **chronic bronchitis.**

*Once thought to be the cause of influenza, which we now know is caused by a virus

Bordetella pertussis. Enters by upper respiratory tract. Cause of **whooping cough** or **pertussis**

Brucella

Very small rods. Inhabit animals, particularly cattle, sheep, goats and swine and are excreted in milk of cattle and goats. All the brucellae seem to be pathogenic for man.

Br. suis.
Found in swine. Cause of a type of **undulant fever.** More common in the United States than in Great Britain

Br. abortus.
Found in cattle. Cause of **undulant fever** or abortus fever. Cause of **abortion in cattle** in Great Britain

Br. melitensis.
Found in goats. Cause of **undulant fever** or Malta fever. Common in Mediterranean countries but not in Great Britain

All the brucellae enter through the mucous membranes of the intestine, either by infected milk or indirectly through personal contact with infected animals. In Great Britain the disease is generally spread through batches of infected milk, though brucellosis is still fairly common in farm hands and veterinary workers. From the intestine the organisms pass into the blood stream, and may be grown from samples of the patient's blood (blood culture). Patients may develop antibodies detectable in serum agglutinin tests, and these tests are carried out on sera of patients with pyrexia of unknown origin.

Pasteurella and Associated Species

Small rods with polar granules. Inhabit insects, particularly fleas and ticks, which pass them on to rodents, which in turn infect other insects. Human beings may become involved in the pasteurellae life cycle if brought in contact with certain insects and certain rodents. Some of the pasteurellae are found in animals (e.g. cats) without any known intervention by insects.

P. pestis.
Inhabits the rat flea, which lives on blood of the plague rats. Other fleas bite the infected rats and then bite men, causing **bubonic** or **pneumonic plague**

P.septica.*
Carried by domestic cats and dogs which transfer the organism by a bite or scratch causing wound infections which are very slow to heal.

*This is not the cause of **cat scratch fever**, which is caused by a virus

In all these infections the organisms usually enter by puncture of the skin, thence via lymphatics to blood stream but they may also be inhaled. This latter is the mode of infection in pneumonic plague.

Francisella tularensis

Inhabits ticks which bite rats and squirrels, which infect other ticks which bite men, causing tularaemia. Unknown in Great Britain, well known in the United States. Tularaemia is generally acquired by persons who handle infected animal carcasses.

Yersinia

Infections due to *Yersinia enterocolitica* affecting first animals (e.g. hares, pigs, sheep) and then man, have been spreading rapidly since 1961. The organism is widespread in the environment, in water, and in small mammals which may be healthy carriers. In man, *Yersinia* is a cause of acute enterocolitis. Infection is thought to occur by the faecal— oral route and to be more common in children and adolescents.

Legionella

Legionella pneumophila infections recognized (and named) after an outbreak of severe pneumonia affecting members attending a meeting of the American Legion in 1976. Since recognized in many countries as a cause of severe pneumonia generally affecting middle-aged men with other pathology.

The causative organism is a poorly staining Gram-indifferent coccobacillus found in soil and water that is transmitted through the air. Many cases have been traced to contaminated humidification of air conditioning systems. At the time of writing there is no evidence that case to case transmission occurs. Primary culture is difficult and cases are often diagnosed by the demonstration of rising levels of specific antibodies. Much research remains to be done on the organism and its relationship to the disease.

Intestinal Organisms

Small rods, sometimes motile, sometimes encapsulated. Widely distributed in nature, in the intestinal tract of man and animals. Some species are pathogenic in the gut; others, e.g. the majority of types of *E. coli*, are normal inhabitants of the gut but may be pathogenic elsewhere in the body. Some, such as *Serratia* and *Enterobacter,* are of low pathogenicity. They are sometimes described as opportunists because they are able to take advantage of diminished immune response and to cause superimposed infection in moist, open wounds, or urinary tract infection in association with poor drainage or irrigation equipment.

Escherichia and klebsiella

These organisms are distinguished from each other by biochemical tests.

Escherichia coli. Found in the urinary tract in pyelitis, pyelonephritis and cystitis. Also found in wounds and may occasionally cause meningitis. Certain types of *E. coli* are associated with neonatal gastroenteritis.

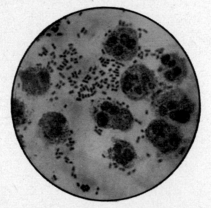

Fig. 34. Deposit from an infected urine showing pus cells and profuse *Escherichia coli* (× 1000).

Klebsiella spp. Commonly found in hospital practice causing wound, urinary, respiratory and other infections. Found in relatively small numbers in the normal intestinal tract. *Klebsiella pneumoniae* (Friedlander's bacillus) is found in the respiratory tract and is said to be responsible for about 3% of cases of pneumonia.

Salmonella
Small motile rods, indistinguishable from *Escherichia* except by biochemical and serological tests and inhabiting the same places. All members are pathogenic.

ENTERIC FEVER GROUP

Salmonella typhi (typhoid bacillus) cause of typhoid fever.

Salm. paratyphi B cause of paratyphoid fever in Great Britain.

Salm. paratyphi A common in Asia.

Salm. paratyphi C uncommon in Great Britain, common in Europe.

These organisms enter the intestine in contaminated food, milk or water. They then pass into the lymphatics, thence to the blood stream and bone marrow, and back to the lymphoid tissue of the reticuloendothelial system. They are excreted in faeces, urine, and possibly vomit.

FOOD POISONING GROUP

A large number of named types exist. Commonly found in Great Britain are, e.g. *Salm. typhimurium, Salm. enteriditis, Salm. dublin.* The organisms enter the intestine in food or drink, and their effects are confined to the intestinal tract.

Shigella

Small rod, indistinguishable from *Escherichia,* but non-motile. The habitat of these organisms is limited to the intestinal tract of man and other primates.

Sh. shiga.	*Sh. flexneri.*	*Sh. sonnei.*	*Sh. boydii.*
Very rare in Great Britain	6 types fairly common in Great Britain	Very common in Great Britain	Several types, rare in Great Britain

The organisms are the cause of *bacillary dysentery*. They are distinguished from other intestinal organisms by biochemical and serological tests. Infection is spread by human carriers and cases. The organisms produce their effect on the mucous membrane of the large intestine. Besides those mentioned above, *Sh. schmitzi, Sh. alkalescens* and *Sh. dispar* are occasionally found in Great Britain. *Sh. sonnei* is usually found in children, and *Sh. flexneri* is common among patients in mental institutions.

Proteus, Pseudomonas and Vibrio

Motile rods which are self-sufficient and independent, inhabiting air, soil and especially water, and found in excreta of man and animals.

Proteus spp. There are four species of *Proteus,* but the one most often found in human infections is *P. mirabilis.* This organism commonly infects the urinary tract and its ability to split urea causes the urine to smell of ammonia. It may also be pathogenic in any site outside the intestinal tract.

Pseudomonas aeruginosa (pyocyanea). This organism takes advantage of diminished natural resistance and thus commonly infects burns, tracheostomies, etc. It will rapidly colonize wet reservoirs such as humidifiers or sink traps. It has a characteristic smell and produces a blue/green pigment which may colour pus.

Vibrio. A comma-shaped motile rod. *Vibrio cholera,* the cause of Asiatic cholera, is pathogenic only to man. Infection is spread by water and the organism affects the intestinal tract only. *Vibrio parahaemolyticus* is a cause of food poisoning associated with eating contaminated shellfish. It is particularly common in Japan but occurs elsewhere.

Campylobacter

Campylobacter species are Gram-negative Vibrio like rods; indeed one variety causing abortion in cattle was classified as a Vibrio until recently. The organisms cause bloody diarrhoea and colic in man. Cases have frequently occurred recently, after eating undercooked poultry or infected milk.

3. BRANCHING BACTERIA AND ACTINOMYCETACEAE

A huge family of organisms which may be Gram-positive, Gram-negative or intermediate. They are distinguished from other bacteria because they branch. They inhabit soil, air, plants and animals and include the streptomyces (source of streptomycin and other antibiotics).

Gram-Positive Members

Club-ended tangled filaments

Anaerobes

Aerobes

Actinomyces israeli.
Method of entry
variable. Causes
chronic granulo-
matous lesions of
jaw, caecum and
appendix, lung etc.

Nocardia madurae.
Cause of the tropical
disease **Madura foot**

Nocardia asteroides.
Causes of **chronic
abscess in lungs and
muscles**

Rudimentary branching

Erysipelothrix rhusiopathiae, or
swine fever bacillus. Enters
through scratch or skin
puncture by some article
infected by rats or by infected
swine. Causes cellulitis of hand
and forearm called **erysipeloid**
seen often in fish porters. When
caught from infected swine
there is usually a severe infection

Actinomyces muris, or
Streptobacillus moniliformis.
Enters through skin by rat bite
or scratch, but may be taken in
infected milk. Causes fever,
rash, endocarditis and
polyarthritis, which is
sometimes called **Haverhill
fever** or **rat-bite fever**

Gram-Negative Members

Bacteroides spp. A large group of non-sporing anaerobic, usually Gram-negative, bacteria. Normal inhabitants of genital and intestinal tracts, but they may cause severe postoperative wound infections, often in association with other organisms, e.g. peritonitis following bowel surgery. *Bacteroides* spp. are the most numerous of the gut commensals.

Fusiform spp. (fusiform bacilli). Fusiform bacilli accompanied by *Borrelia vincentii* (page 154) are found in smears of mouth, gums and fauces in the ulcerative gingivitis known as *Vincent's angina*.

Mycoplasma. Characterized by absence of cell wall and therefore of indefinite shapes and sizes. Aerobic, difficult to grow. Group also known as PPLO (pleuro-pneumonia-like organisms), so called because they resemble the organisms which cause pleuro-pneumonia in cattle. Found on mucous membranes of eyes and genitalia.

  Mycoplasma pneumoniae causes primary atypical pneumonia.

4. ACID-FAST DIVISION

Mycobacterium

Slender rods, are enveloped with unsaponifiable wax which renders the organisms difficult to stain by Gram's method. After staining by hot carbol fuchsin, the organisms are stain-fast, resisting decolorization with alcohols and strong mineral acids. Non-pathogenic forms are widely distributed in nature, e.g. *Myco. smegmatis, Myco. butyricum.*

PATHOGENIC

Myco. leprae. Cannot be cultured and is not pathogenic for animals. Cause of **leprosy** which is diagnosed micro- scopically from scrapings or sections of material from patients	*Myco. tuberculosis,* or tubercle bacilli	A number of strains of low pathogenicity, e.g. *Myco. balnei* cause of **swimming pool granuloma**

Human type; cause of **pulmonary tuberculosis**	Bovine type; cause of **body and glandular tuberculosis**

Mycobacterium tuberculosis is a slow growing organism. If present in sufficiently large numbers it may be seen on direct microscopy but before a laboratory diagnosis of tuberculosis can be confirmed or eliminated it has to be grown on a special culture medium. This may take as long as six to eight weeks.

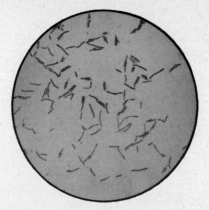

Fig. 35. Culture smear of *Mycobacterium tuberculosis* (× 1500). Note characteristic slightly curved, delicate bacilli.

5. SPIROCHAETES

Slender rods, moving by flexing and corkscrew motion. Visualized by dark ground illumination of the microscope field because they are difficult or impossible to stain by usual methods. Non-pathogenic spirochaetes are found in the mouth, on gums and the genitalia.

PATHOGENIC

Leptospira.
Corkscrew-shaped with hooked ends

Many species, e.g. *L. icterohaemorrhagiae.* Cause of **infectious jaundice or Weil's disease.** Carried by rats and enters through contamination of damaged skin or mucous membrane, associated with sewer workers

Treponema.
Very delicate regular coils

Trep. pallidum
Cause of **syphilis.** Enters through mucous membrane of genitourinary tract, mouth, or other direct contact site

Trep. pertenue.
Cause of **yaws,** in tropical countries. Spread by direct contact with skin lesions

Borrelia.
Large, wormlike

Borrelia recurrentis and *Borrelia duttoni* are carried by lice or ticks to human hosts who develop relapsing fever (tropical countries). *Borrelia vincentii* (or Vincent's spirochaete) accompanied by *Fusiformis* sp. are found in the ulcerative condition of the mouth and gums known as **Vincent's angina**

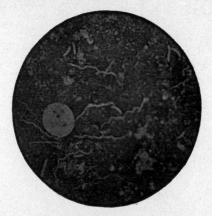

Fig. 36. Direct smear from the throat of a patient with Vincent's angina. Note the characteristic spirochaetes and fusiform bacilli (× 1000).

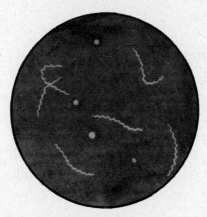

Fig. 37. *Trepenoma pallidum* from a primary syphilitic lesion (× 1000).

6. RICKETTSIAE

Rickettsiae are grouped between bacteria and viruses. Specimens are tested for Rickettsiae in the virology laboratory (see Chapter 10).

7. VIRUSES

The many varieties of virus and the diseases that they cause are outlined in Chapter 10.

Summary of Bacterial Transmission

Pathogen	Portal of Entry	Clinical Disease	Route of Exit	Usual Source of Infection	Accommodation
Streptococcus (beta haemolytic streptococcus Group A)	Upper respiratory tract	Tonsillitis	Respiratory secretions	Human cases and throat and nasal carriers	Single room for 48 hours Systemic penicillin then ward if apyrexial
		Otitis media	Aural and respiratory secretions		
		Meningitis	None		
		Secondary pneumonia	Sputum		
	Any route, usually upper respiratory tract	Scarlet fever	Secretions from lesions and respiratory		
	Skin	Erysipelas, cellulitis			
		Wound infection	Pus from lesions		
	Locally at placental site	Puerperal sepsis	Lochia		
	Possible sequelae to listed infections	Rheumatic fever	None		Ward
		Acute nephritis	None		Ward
Streptococcus pneumoniae (pneumococcus)	Respiratory tract	Pneumonia	Sputum	Commensal organism, opportunist, i.e. infection only when contributory factor, e.g. damaged mucosa, congestion	Ward
		Sinusitis	Nasal secretions		
		Otitis media	Aural and respiratory nasal secretions		
	Middle ear, sinuses	Meningitis	None		Ward
	Conjunctiva	Conjunctivitis	Conjunctival secretions		Ward

Pathogen	Portal of Entry	Clinical Disease	Route of Exit	Usual Source of Infection	Accommodation
Streptococcus faecalis	Gut lesions to blood stream	Subacute bacterial endocarditis	None	Gut	Ward
	Contact transmission	Wound infection	Pus from lesions		Ward
	Via urethra	Urinary tract infection	Urine		Ward
Staphylococcus aureus (*Staphylococcus pyogenes*, coagulase positive *Staphylococcus*)	Local, skin	Boils, carbuncles, whitlows, impetigo, wound infections	Pus from lesions	Human cases and carriers *Transmission by hands, equipment, bedding and clothing*	Single room unless very minor lesion
	Surgery	Deep abscesses	Pus after incision		
	Blood stream	Osteomyelitis	Pus after incision		
	Respiratory tract	Otitis media	Discharge from ear		
		Pneumonia	Sputum		
	Ingestion of infected food, carbohydrate, e.g. trifle, custard	Toxic vomiting (food poisoning)	Faeces and vomit for a few hours. N.B. any remaining food dangerous	Enterotoxin strain in staff handling food, e.g. septic finger	Ward
	From skin or deep infection	Septicaemia	None (excluding initial lesion)		

Organism	Mode of spread	Disease	Infectious material	Source	Isolation
Neisseria gonorrhoeae (*gonococcus*)	Direct spread during coitus	Gonorrhoea ♂Urethritis, epididymitis, prostatis ♀Urethritis, cervicitis, vulvovaginitis, salpingitis	Discharges from urethra and vagina	Human cases	Single room for 48 hours; systemic penicillin then ward
	Blood stream from primary	Arthritis	None		Ward
	Eye	Ophthalmia neonatorum	Conjunctival secretions	Maternal vaginal discharge	Single room
Neisseria meningitidis (*meningococcus*)	Respiratory tract	Meningitis (cerebrospinal fever) Septicaemia with rash and arthritis	Nasal secretions Skin lesions	Human nasopharyngeal carriers, close contact transmission	Single room until nasopharyngeal secretions negative (usually 48 hours) then ward
	Eye	Ophthalmitis	Discharge from eyes		
Corynebacterium diphtheriae	Respiratory tract	Diphtheria Organism infects nasal cavity, pharynx, tonsils, larynx, trachea; rarely conjunctiva, wound or vagina: toxin absorbed from theses sites causes the disease	Respiratory tract secretions	Cases, convalescent cases, and carriers (usually in nose or throat)	Isolation unit until 2 negative nasal and 2 negative throat swabs Usually up to 14 days
	Local		From secretions		

Pathogen	Portal of Entry	Clinical Disease	Route of Exit	Usual Source of Infection	Accommodation
Mycobacterium tuberculosis (tubercle bacillus)	Respiratory tract Ingestion	Tuberculosis (a) Pulmonary (b) Cervical glands (c) Alimentary tract	Sputum Discharging sinus Faeces	Open cases Infected milk Infected or swallowed sputum	(a) Tuberculosis unit or single room until negative culture (b) and (c) Preferably single room
	Lymphatic/blood stream spread of primary	Miliary tuberculosis Meningitis Bone + joint lesions } Kidney lesions Testicular lesions Fallopian tube plus uterine lesions	Any open lesion Urine Menstrual fluid		
Mycobacterium leprae	Direct contact, probably through skin or mucous membrane	Leprosy (a) Cutaneous (nodular) (b) Neural (anaesthetic)	Skin lesions	Close, continuous contact with an open case, e.g. familial	Ward

Organism	Transmission	Disease	Specimen	Source / Reservoir	Isolation / Nursing
Bacillus anthracis	Direct contact Inhalation of spores	Anthrax (a) Cutaneous (b) Pulmonary (wood sorter's disease)	Skin lesions Sputum	Infected animal hides and furs, etc.	Isolation unit or 'strict isolation' in single room. Rarely transmitted man to man, spore contaminated items may remain infective for years
Bacillus cereus	Ingestion	Diarrhoeal gastroenteritis	Faeces	Infected food, typically rice that has been partially cooked some time before final cooking	Ward
Clostridium tetani	Injury, usually a puncture wound	Tetanus Symptoms due to powerful neurotoxin	Discharging wound	Soil containing spores from animal faeces	Usually non-infective. Single room required for other medical reasons
Clostridium welchii (*perfringens*) and related strains	Contamination of devitalized muscle	Gas gangrene Symptoms due to toxaemia, may lead to septicaemia	Discharge from lesion	Present in faeces of normal man and animals	Hyperbaric O_2 unit Ward
Heat resistant Type A strains	Ingestion	Food poisoning diarrhoea		Contaminated food	Ward
Clostridium botulinum	Ingestion	Botulism. A pure toxaemia, about 70% mortality	None. Organism grows in food, not in intestine	Rare. Home canned vegetables or home cured meat	Ward Assisted respiration

Pathogen	Portal of Entry	Clinical Disease	Route of Exit	Usual Source of Infection	Accommodation
Actinomyces israeli	Ingestion	Actinomycosis Subacute or chronic granulomatous disease Suppuration and fistulae, usually cervicofacial, abdominal or thoracic	Discharge from lesions	Endogenous. Normal mouth flora, opportunist organism	Ward
Treponema pallidum	(a) Placenta	Congenital syphilis	Secretions of respiratory tract (nasal + lung lesion)	Syphilitic mother	Single room for 48 hrs Systemic penicillin then ward
	(b) Skin or mucous membrane Via blood stream	Primary syphilis (chancre) Secondary syphilis	Discharge from chancre Discharge from surface lesions e.g. mouth ulcer	Direct contact during coitus Contact with infected lesions, e.g. coitus, kissing, mouth care	Ward
		Tertiary syphilis Gummata, dementia, meningo and cardiovascular tabes	None other than discharge from surface gumma		
Leptospira icterohaemorrhagiae	Ingestion, or by abrasions in skin or mucous membrane	Weil's disease (spirochaetal jaundice). Common in sewer workers	Urine	Rats spread organism and excrete it in urine. Contaminated water	Ward

Organism	Mode of spread	Disease	Infective material	Source	Accommodation
Borrelia vincentii	Mouth normal flora, opportunist organism	Vincent's angina, with a fusiform bacillus	Respiratory secretions	Human carriers or cases	Ward
Escherichia coli	Via urethra Perforated gut Contact transmission	Urinary tract infection Peritonitis Infection of wounds, burns	Urine None Discharge from lesions	Gut and faecal contamination	Ward
Enteropathogenic strains	Ingestion	Diarrhoea in infants and the very old	Faeces	Human carriers or cases	Isolation unit or single room
Salmonella Enteric fever group: *S. typhi, S. paratyphi*	Ingestion	Enteric fever (typhoid and paratyphoid)	All secretions during septicaemia for first two weeks: faeces, urine	Human carriers or cases via water or food	Single room
Food poisoning group: *Salmonella typhimurium* and over 800 others		Gastroenteritis	Vomit and faeces	Human or animal carriers or cases via food	
Shigella, numerous types, e.g. *S. sonnei*	Ingestion	Bacillary dysentery	Faeces	Human carriers or cases	Single room
Proteus mirabilis	Via urethra Contact transmission	Urinary tract infection Wound and respiratory infections	Urine Discharges	Gut, nasal, external ear carriers	Depends on the extent and severity of the infection

Pathogen	Portal of Entry	Clinical Disease	Route of Exit	Usual Source of Infection	Accommodation
Pseudomonas aeruginosa (*Pseudomonas pyocyanea*)	Contact transmission	Infection in tissues damaged by disease, accident or surgery, e.g. bronchiectasis, burns, tracheostomy, surgical wound and urinary tract infection	Secretions and discharges	Organism often present in the gut Reservoirs in wet situations, e.g. humidifiers, sink traps, flower water etc.	Depends on the extent and severity of the infection
Klebsiella spp.	Some strains normally present in respiratory tract	Respiratory tract infections, e.g. pneumonia	Nasal and bronchial secretions	Endogenous. Easily transmissable via wet media, hands, instruments	Depends on the extent and severity of the infection
	Contact transmission	Wound infections	Discharges		
	Via urethra	Urinary tract infection	Urine		
Vibrio cholera	Ingestion	Asiatic cholera Diarrhoea and vomiting Affects intestinal tract only	Faeces and vomit	Human cases or carriers via contaminated water or food	Isolation unit
Campylobacter	Ingestion	Bloody diarrhoea	Faeces (probably not usually transmitted by cases or carriers)	Infected food of animal origin, often undercooked poultry	Ward

Organism	Route of entry	Disease	Method of spread	Source / reservoir	Accommodation
Haemophilus influenzae	Respiratory tract	Secondary respiratory infections; infects mucosa damaged by influenza virus / Meningitis in children / Septic arthritis	Respiratory secretions / None / None	Often found as normal mouth flora, some cause infection	Ward
	Conjunctiva	Conjunctivitis	Conjunctival secretions		
Haemophilus ducreyi	Direct contact during coitus	Soft chancre (chancroid)	Discharge from chancre	Human case, intercourse	
Bordetella pertussis	Respiratory tract	Whooping cough	Respiratory secretions	Cases	Isolation unit
Brucella abortus *Brucella melitensis*	Ingestion	Brucellosis (undulant and Malta fevers)	Usually none, occasionally in urine	Unpasteurized cow's or goat's milk	Ward
Legionella pneumophila	Respiratory tract	Legionnaire's disease (severe pneumonia)	Sputum (no evidence of transmissibility case to case)	Evidence incomplete but many cases associated with contaminated air conditioning systems	Ward, but keep away from other patients
Candida albicans (Monilia)	Damaged tissues	Candidiasis: Mouth (thrush) / Skin, septic fingers / Vagina / Systemic	Exudates	Often found in normal mouth, vagina, intestines. Opportunist organism	Ward except for very severe infection, then single room

10 A Guide to Common Viruses

Infection

Many infections are known to be due to viruses; others are believed to be when no bacterial source of infection can be demonstrated in an obviously transmissible disease. Virus infections are common and most are mild (e.g. colds). Some are 'silent' and the virus multiplies in the body, usually without causing disease (e.g. cytomegalovirus), some cause latent infection (e.g. herpes simplex), a few cause very severe or fatal illness (e.g. smallpox).

Many viruses enter the body by inhalation (e.g. influenza, measles), others gain entry by ingestion (e.g. poliomyelitis), or inoculation (e.g. hepatitis B), all spread locally directly to the tissues and some are disseminated widely via the blood stream. Viruses invade living cells and 'take over' the cell metabolic processes to reproduce themselves; the cell usually dies and releases the virus particles but it may survive and carry the virus as in latent infections. Certain viruses can induce changes in the genetic material of cells causing them to undergo malignant transformation.

Defence mechanisms

Cells invaded and infected by a virus produce a protein substance, *interferon*, in the acute stage of the disease. This is released and temporarily protects other cells which take it up, from infection. Viral antigens stimulate the production of antibodies which are carried in the patient's serum and neutralize any subsequent invasion by the same virus, i.e. the patient becomes immune to that virus. Specific immunity, of which circulating antibody is one manifestation, persists often for many years, but may gradually decrease to a level where the patient is again susceptible or partially susceptible to infection. For example, herpes zoster (shingles) occurring in an adult is due to the same virus which caused his childhood attack of varicella (chickenpox); the recrudescent infection occurs when the immunity level has decreased.

Destruction of viruses

Most viruses are killed by exposure to heat such as boiling for a few minutes, but survive storage at temperatures as low as −70°C. Their ability to withstand drying is very variable but all are thought to be sensitive to ultra-violet light. In general terms viruses can be destroyed by the action of aldehydes, chlorine, iodine and hydrogen peroxide; some are completely resistant to the phenolic group of disinfectants; a chlorine derivative, e.g. Chloros, hypochlorite, is commonly used for disinfection purposes. The advice of a virologist should be taken in outbreaks of infection since different viruses vary in their reaction to chemicals.

Only certain viruses contain lipid and the fact that lipid-containing viruses are inactivated by ether or chloroform is used in the laboratory identification and classification of viruses.

Laboratory identification

Light microscopy. Inclusion bodies may be present in tissue cells as a result of virus infection. They are seen as clumps of virus particles within the cytoplasm, e.g. trachoma, or as an eosinophilic mass in the cell nucleus, e.g. herpes.

Electron microscopy. Using a beam of electrons focussed by magnets structures as small as 0.5 nm can be resolved, and the characteristic morphology of different groups of viruses recognized.

Antibody. Recent infection is indicated either by a rise in antibody titre or by the presence of IgM class antibodies to the infecting virus. Two blood samples are required to demonstrate a rising titre, one taken during the acute phase of the illness and another about fourteen days later.

Culture. Viruses can be grown in the laboratory by inoculating:

1. A tissue culture of cells grown in a single layer on the wall of a glass test tube.
2. Chick embryos in fertile hens' eggs.
3. Laboratory animals.

Some viral antigens may be identified directly without culturing the virus by serological tests, e.g. hepatitis B virus.

Classification.

Viruses are grouped acording to their nucleic acid, size, symmetry, structure, sensitivity to ether and by the diseases which they cause. Further classification is by serological specificity and cultural characteristics.

ADENOVIRUS GROUP

DNA viruses Icosahedral. 75 nm

Diagnostic material: Mouth washings, throat swabs, faeces, conjunctival swabs (in eye disease)

There are 31 serotypes in this group; the viruses attack lymphoid tissue and may cause:

Pharyngitis	**Conjunctivitis**	**Mesenteric adenitis**
	May be spread by eye instruments	Diarrhoea

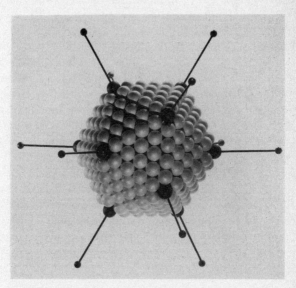

Fig. 38. Model of adenovirus showing its 'antennae'.

HERPESVIRUS GROUP

DNA viruses. Icosahedral with an outer envelope. 120–200 nm

Diagnostic material: Vesicle fluid, skin swabs, saliva, conjuctival fluid/scrapings (eye cases); urine (*cytomegalovirus*); cervical, vaginal swabs (*herpes genitalis*)

Chemotherapy: Acylovir and adenine arabinoside have been used for systemic infections and idoxuridine for superficial infections

These viruses are common in man, often causing symptomless and latent infections, e.g. most adults have antibodies to both herpes simplex and cytomegalovirus without symptoms or history of infection.

Herpes simplex. Primary infection in early childhood is often mild or unrecognized, but may cause gingivostomatitis or conjunctivitis. Other primary infections are *herpes genitalis,* i.e. *Herpesvirus hominis* Type II (venereal transmission), whitlow from contact during nursing care, severe generalized neonatal infection which may be acquired at birth. 'Cold sores' are common recrudescent episodes of infection, the virus is thought to remain latent in the trigeminal nerve ganglion between attacks and to be reactivated by non-specific stimuli, e.g. sun, colds. Recurrent infection of the eye causes dendritic corneal ulcers. Encephalitis is a rare complication generally of latent infection.

Varicella/zoster. *Varicella* (chickenpox) is the primary infection. The virus then remains latent in nerve ganglia; when the level of immunity decreases it may be reactivated, resulting in an attack of *zoster* (shingles). Zoster is not

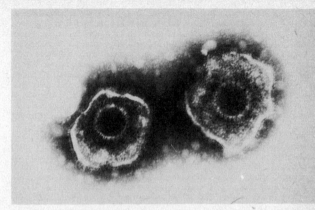

Fig. 39. Two Herpesivirus particles from a vesicle of a patient suffering from chickenpox (× 60 000).

usually acquired by contact with another case or with varicella, but it may cause varicella in susceptible persons, e.g. a nurse who has not had chickenpox. Patients undergoing immunosuppressive therapy are particularly susceptible to varicella/zoster.

Cytomegalovirus. Commonly symptomless but it may cause severe generalized neonatal infection, or an illness similar to glandular fever in adults. Generalized infection may occur when immunity is impaired by immunosuppressive drugs.

Epstein-Barr virus. This virus causes infectious mononucleosis (glandular fever). It is also found associated with Burkitt's lymphoma although its exact role in the development of this tumour is uncertain.

POXVIRUS GROUP

DNA viruses. Brick-shaped, complex structure. 200–300 nm.

Diagnostic material: Vesicle fluid, crusts, scrapings from maculo-papules

This virus group includes:

Variola	**Variola minor**	**Vaccinia**	
(smallpox)	(alastrim)	Used for smallpox vaccine	Many animal pox viruses

Variola (smallpox) is a severe disease with a high mortality rate in unvaccinated persons. A milder form of the disease known as alastrim occurred in some parts of the world. Smallpox vaccine is prepared from the closely related, but much less virulent, vaccinia virus. Complete immunity lasts for about three years after vaccination but partial protection which modifies the severity of the disease lasts for considerably longer. When a case of smallpox is detected the patient is nursed in strict isolation and every effort made to trace all contacts immediately and place them in quarantine; vaccine has to be given early in the incubation period, which averages 12 days, to be effective. Patients with smallpox are strictly isolated, usually in a special unit, because although the main route of infection is by respiratory spread, the virus can survive for years in disseminated, dried skin scabs.

In 1980 the WHO announced that following an intensive programme smallpox had been eradicated worldwide. The need for vaccination is now confined to a few health-care workers, e.g. doctors and nurses working in designated smallpox units. Large supplies of vaccine are kept as a precaution against the unlikely re-emergence of the disease.

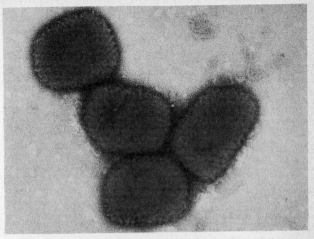

Fig. 40. Smallpox virus particles from a vesicle (× 60 000).

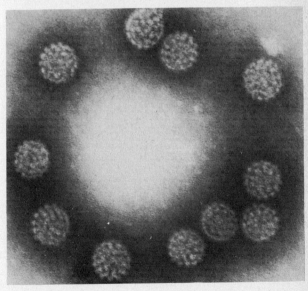

Fig. 41. Wart virus particles (× 150 000) from a plantar wart.

MYXOVIRUS GROUP

RNA viruses. Helical. 80–120 nm

Diagnostic material: Mouth washings, throat swabs

Influenza A virus is the principal cause of epidemic influenza.

Influenza B virus causes smaller epidemics and outbreaks.

Both viruses attack and desquamate the epithelium of the respiratory tract leaving it susceptible to secondary bacterial invasion, e.g. staphylococcal infection.

Influenza C virus rarely causes clinical infection.

Influenza virus vaccines are available, they give some protection but are not always effective because of the multiplicity of strains. The viruses, particularly influenza A, develop variant strains. Occasionally completely new strains emerge to which the whole world population is susceptible; a pandemic then occurs. Influenza spreads very rapidly, the incubation period is short (two days) and the speed of spread of a new strain often makes it impossible to prepare enough vaccine in time to protect everybody. It is usual therefore to restrict protection to, for example, people with chronic respiratory disease and essential hospital and public service staff. Vaccine must be given before an epidemic starts since antibodies are not formed immediately.

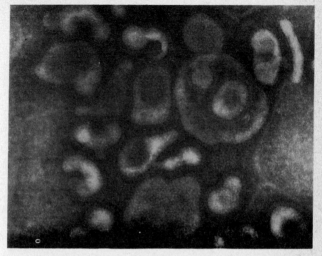

Fig. 42. Influenza virus (× 75 000) grown in a fertile **egg for vaccine** production.

PARAMYXOVIRUS GROUP

RNA viruses. Helical. 90–250 nm

Diagnostic material: Mouth washings, nasal secretions, throat swabs (parainfluenza)

Parotitis (mumps)	Measles	Parainfluenzae Croup <5 years	Respiratory syncytial virus (RSV) Bronchiolitis in young children

Measles. In the United Kingdom and other countries where living conditions are good the disease is usually mild, but in countries where nutrition levels and living conditions are poor, measles is a serious disease and frequently fatal. In

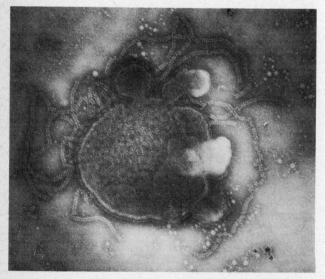

Fig. 43. Paramyxovirus; a disrupted mumps particle showing fragments of internal nucleocapsid (×60000).

the United Kingdom immunization is given in childhood to avoid the complications, e.g. respiratory tract infections, encephalitis, which occur in some cases. When a child develops measles after admission to a nursery or hospital ward it is usual to protect susceptible contacts by administering gamma-globulin. Gamma-globulin is prepared from pooled human plasma (i.e. from many donors) which contains antibody to measles because most adults have had the disease. This is an example of passive immunization. Sub-acute sclerosing pan-encephalitis is a late, rare and fatal complication of past measles virus infection.

RUBELLA VIRUS

RNA virus. About 60 nm
Diagnostic material: Blood
Rubella (German measles) is a mild illness but if the disease is transmitted to a pregnant woman during the first four months of pregnancy the virus may cause congenital defects in the fetus, e.g. deafness, cataract, heart defects. In the United Kingdom rubella virus vaccine is given to 12–13-year-old girls, the aim being to protect against rubella before childbearing age without attempting to prevent cases in children. It may also be offered to women of childbearing age shown by serological tests to be non-immune. Pregnancy should be avoided for two months after vaccination to ensure that there is no possibility of fetal infection due to the attenuated virus.

CORONAVIRUS GROUP

RNA viruses. 100 nm
   These viruses cause respiratory disease which is generally mild.

VIRAL HEPATITIS

Hepatitis A: RNA virus, 28 nm
Hepatitis B: DNA virus. 42 nm
Diagnostic material: Blood

Virus A (*infectious hepatitis*) is transmitted from person to person by faecally contaminated water or food. The disease is endemic in most countries and has an incubation period of about 30 days, it spreads easily in close contact situations, e.g. families, nursery schools. No active immunization is available against infectious hepatitis but human immunoglobulin is given for short-term passive immunity (3–6 months).

Virus B (*serum hepatitis*) may be transmitted from person to person by inoculation of infected blood, e.g. from a contaminated hypodermic syringe and needle, medical and laboratory equipment, tattooing and acupuncture. It is also transmitted between sexual partners especially male homosexuals. It can be transmitted by blood or blood products.

The incubation period of hepatitis B is 40 to 180 days and the disease is differentiated from hepatitis A by testing for antigen in the blood serum. Hepatitis B surface antigen (Australia antigen or HBs Ag) can be detected only in the serum of patients who are incubating or actually have acute hepatitis B, or in jaundice-free persons who still carry the antigen from a previous often unrecognized infection. The silent carriage rate amongst the indigenous population in Great Britain is about 1 in 1000. It is known to be greater in high risk groups, e.g. drug addicts, male homosexuals and many overseas populations. Most carriers of the virus remain healthy but a few develop chronic active hepatitis

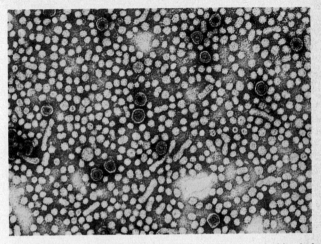

Fig. 44. Hepatitis B surface antigen (HBs Ag) purified from the blood of a carrier. The large particles with an inner core are complete infectious virions ($\times 60\,000$).

and cirrhosis. Chronic infections with hepatitis B virus may be responsible for the development of hepatoma.

Specific human immunoglobulin gives passive immunity and may be administered following accidental inoculations of infected blood. A vaccine prepared from inactivated HBs Ag has been shown to give good protection.

Non-A, non-B hepatitis

The use of serological tests to identify cases of acute hepatitis A and B has shown that most acute viral hepatitis in tropical countries is not due to either of these viruses. The so far unidentified viruses responsible have been labelled non-A, non-B hepatitis viruses. In Western countries they are a cause of post-transfusion hepatitis and are also responsible for some sporadic cases of acute hepatitis in adults.

PICORNAVIRUS GROUP

RNA viruses. Small icosahedral. 26 nm

Diagnostic material: Faeces, throat swabs, cerebrospinal fluid, nasal secretions, mouth washings, depending on clinical symptoms

Rhinoviruses. 50 serotypes. Main cause of common colds.

Enteroviruses. Poliovirus, Echo virus, Coxsackie virus, are ingested, multiply in the alimentary tract and spread from the gut to tissues and organs via the blood stream. Virus is excreted in the faeces.

Poliovirus causes poliomyelitis, but symptomless intestinal infections are common. There are three serological types of poliovirus; attenuated strains of each type are incorporated in trivalent oral poliovaccine. The use of vaccine has virtually eliminated poliomyelitis in many countries. Immunization with poliovaccine should be given in childhood (page 49), but the vaccine should also be given to adults who may be exposed to the virus, e.g. in hospital or when travelling to countries where poliomyelitis is still common.

Coxsackie viruses cause 'hand, foot and mouth' disease, herpangina, Bornholm disease (epidemic myalgia), myocarditis and pericarditis.

Echo and Coxsackie viruses occasionally cause aseptic meningitis and all are common where living conditions and hygiene are poor, though most infections are symptomless.

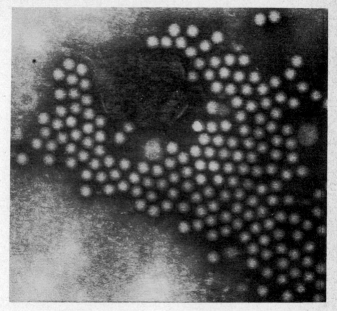

Fig. 45. Poliovirus particles in a purified vaccine (× 100 000).

REOVIRUS GROUP

RNA virus. 60–66 nm. Icosahedral
Diagnostic material: Faeces

Rotavirus, so called because it looks like a wheel, has recently been identified in outbreaks of gastroenteritis and febrile diarrhoea in infants and young children. Infection occurs most commonly during the winter months and in children under three years old. The virus is transmissable by the faecal–oral route and usually causes only mild to moderately severe disease. Gastroenteritis in children and adults may also be caused by a number of other smaller viruses.

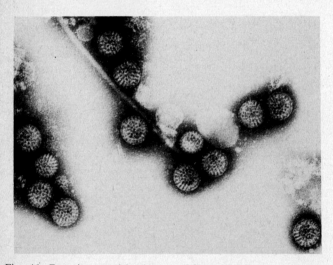

Fig. 46. Rotavirus particles in a partially purified faecal suspension (× 100 000).

ARBOVIRUS GROUP

RNA viruses. 20–150 nm
Diagnostic material: Blood
Important diseases caused include:

Yellow fever   **Encephalitis**   **Systemic febrile disease**

About 50 serotypes cause disease in man. The hosts are birds and small mammals and the virus is transmitted to man by the bite of infected arthropods, i.e. mosquito, tick, sandfly. The diseases are common in many parts of the world though not in the United Kingdom. There is a highly effective attenuated virus vaccine against Yellow fever.

ARENOVIRUS GROUP

RNA viruses. 70–150 nm
Diagnostic material: Blood, throat washings

Lassa fever is an acute haemorrhagic virus disease with a high mortality, first recognized in West Africa in 1969. In endemic areas the virus is transmitted to man in food contaminated by the urine or saliva of an infected rat (*Mastomys natalensis*). Person-to-person transmission is by close contact with the blood, pharyngeal secretions or urine of an infected patient. Immune plasma has been used in treatment.

A similar disease is caused by Marburg and Ebola viruses. They are closely related to one another but are not Arenoviruses. Both are found in tropical Africa and have unknown animal reservoirs.

Modern air travel increases the risk of tropical fevers such as Lassa fever and Marburg disease reaching this country. Patients are nursed in strict isolation and only in scheduled units.

RHABDOVIRUS GROUP

RNA viruses. Bullet-shaped, helical. 37–60 nm
Diagnostic material: Saliva, cerebrospinal fluid, urine

Rabies virus is transmitted from infected dogs, cats, bats, or carnivorous wild animals in the saliva, by biting. Rabies is worldwide except for a few countries like the U.K. where it has been eradicated. The virus spreads from the wound to the central nervous system via nerve tissue and the disease is fatal. The long incubation period (usually 4–12 weeks) makes prophylactic active immunization after exposure possible. A combination of anti-rabies vaccine (active immunization) and heterologous anti-rabies serum or human anti-rabies immunoglobulin (passive immunization) is usually given. Modern vaccines prepared from tissue-culture grown virus are potent and safe.

RICKETTSIAE

Rickettsiae are grouped between viruses and bacteria. Like viruses they multiply only within living cells, but like bacteria contain both RNA and DNA. They can be seen with a light microscope although slightly smaller than bacteria.

The group includes:

R. prowazeki	*R. mooseri*	*R. orientalis*	*R. rickettsi*	*C. burneti*
Typhus fever	Murine typhus	Tsutsuga-mushi fever	Rocky mountain spotted fever	Q fever
Louse-borne	Flea-borne	Mite-borne	Tick-borne	

Epidemic typhus fever is associated with very poor, overcrowded living conditions and is transmitted by the victim scratching infected louse faeces into the skin. It is an epidemic disease, control measures are directed towards eliminating lice; vaccine is available.

Q fever is primarily a disease of large domestic animals, transmitted to man in the milk of infected cows or sheep and by inhalation of dust contaminated by placentae, fetal membranes and fluid after the birth of a calf or lamb to an infected animal. The patient may have atypical pneumonia and very occasionally subacute endocarditis if the heart valves are already damaged.

CHLAMYDIAE

Chlamydiae are grouped between viruses and bacteria. They multiply only within living cells as do viruses, but like bacteria contain both RNA and DNA, can be visualized with a light microscope and measure 250–450 nm.

Psittacosis (ornithosis)	Lympho-granuloma venereum	TRIC agents	Non-specific urethritis and cervicitis

TRIC (trachoma–inclusion conjunctivitis) agents are widespread in tropical countries and associated with poor living conditions and lack of hygiene. The organisms are by contact, contaminated communal possessions and flies, and are a common cause of blindness. In temperate climates they are the commonest cause of non-specific urethritis and cervicitis and sometimes cause conjunctivitis.

Summary of Viral Transmission

Virus	Entry Route	Disease	Exit Route	Usual Source of Infection	Accommodation
Pox group Variola Variola minor	Inhalation	Smallpox	Respiratory secretions vesicle fluid. Dried scabs may remain infectious for years	Cases	Designated isolation unit until scabs have gone. Average 2–3 weeks
Vaccinia	Skin inoculation against smallpox		Exudate	Infected calf lymph i.e. smallpox vaccine	Ward except in cases of severe generalized rash
Adenovirus group 31 serological types	Inhalation Contact Ingestion	Pharyngitis Conjunctivitis Mesenteric adenitis Diarrhoea	Respiratory secretions Conjunctival secretions Faeces	Cases Contact, eye instruments	Avoid overcrowding
Herpes group Herpes simplex I	Contact	**Primary** Usually early in life (a) symptomless (b) gingivostomatitis (c) conjunctivitis Whitlow	Secretions and exudates	Cases	Avoid contact with infants and patients with eczema
Herpes simplex II	Inoculation Contact	Herpes genitalis	Venereal transmission	Cases	
Herpes I and II		**Recurrent** Cold sores Keratoconjunctivitis Encephalitis		Autogenous	

Virus	Entry Route	Disease	Exit Route	Usual Source of Infection	Accommodation
Varicella zoster	Inhalation	Primary chickenpox	Saliva. Skin lesions	Cases	Isolate for 7 days from rash appearing
	Virus latent in nerve	Recurrent shingles		Autogenous	Segregate from non-immune to varicella
Cytomegalovirus	Blood stream	**Neonatal** generalized infection	Saliva Urine	In utero from mother	
		Adult— (a) Inapparent glandular fever type (b) General infection in lowered resistance, e.g. immunosuppressions		Opportunist organism, most adults are symptomless, latent carriers	
Epstein-Barr (EB)	Mouth	Glandular fever	Throat secretions	Probably close contact with case or carrier, e.g. kissing	Avoid close contact
Myxovirus group Influenza A Influenza B	**Myxovirus group** Inhalation	Epidemic influenza Outbreaks of influenza	Droplets of saliva	Cases	Single room until temperature normal for 48 hours
Influenza C		Very occasionally pathogenic			

Paramyxovirus group Parainfluenza, I, II, III, IV	Inhalation	Croup (<5 years)	Droplet infection	Cases	Segregate from babies
Respiratory syncytial virus	Inhalation	Bronchiolitis (< 5 years) usually <1 year	Droplet infection	Cases	Segregate from babies
Mumps	Mouth	Mumps	Saliva		Single room for 7 days
Measles	Inhalation	Measles	Droplet infection		Single room until rash fades +2 days
Rubella	Inhalation	German measles	Droplet infection	Cases and congenital cases	Avoid contact with susceptible women in early pregnancy
Virus hepatitis Virus A	Ingestion	Infectious hepatitis	Faeces, urine	Close contact with cases Contaminated water, food and sometimes shellfish	Preferably single room
Virus B	Parenteral inoculation Probably sometimes by injection	Serum hepatitis	Blood. Possibly other bodily excretions and secretions	Contact with infected blood via needles, blood transfusions, communal syringes tattooing, etc. Sexual partners	Single room if bleeding

Virus	Entry Route	Disease	Exit Route	Usual Source of Infection	Accommodation
Coronavirus group	Inhalation	Respiratory disease	Droplet infection	Cases	Single room during acute phase (assisted respiration may be required if respiratory muscles are involved in poliomyelitis)
Picornavirus group					
Rhinoviruses 50 serotypes	Inhalation	Common colds	Respiratory secretions	Cases	
Enteroviruses	Ingestion Multiply in the alimentary tract Spread from gut to tissues, CNS or organs via the blood stream	Often symptomless Poliomyelitis Aseptic meningitis			
(a) Poliovirus			Faeces	Cases	
(b) Echovirus			Pharyngeal secretions	Poor hygiene and living conditions	
(c) Coxsackie virus A		Hand, foot, and mouth disease Herpangina Aseptic meningitis		Symptom free infections	
Coxsackie virus B		Bornholm disease Myocarditis, pericarditis Aseptic meningitis			
Reovirus group					
Rotavirus	Ingestion	Gastroenteritis <3 years	Faeces	Contaminated food/milk	Segregate from <3 years
Arbovirus group About 50 serotypes cause disease in man	Inoculation	Yellow fever Systemic febrile disease Encephalitis (not UK)	Blood	Birds and mammals via bite of mosquito, tick or sandfly	Mosquito nets

					Designated isolation unit
Arenovirus group Lassa fever virus	Probably ingestion/inhalation	Lassa fever	Blood Urine Pharyngeal secretions	Food and environ-ment contamina-ted by tropical rat urine/saliva Cases	Isolation unit for duration of illness
Rhabdovirus group	Inoculation Spread to CNS via nerves	Rabies (fatal acute disease of CNS)	Saliva Urine	Dogs, cats, bats, carnivorous wild animals (UK free from rabies due to quarantine)	
Papovavirus group Wart virus	Inoculation	Common warts Venereal warts	Material from wart	Cases	
Rickettsiae R. prowazeki	Inoculation (often from infected louse faeces by scratching)	Epidemic typhus fever	Infection of another louse which bites the patient	Alimentary tract of infected lice	
R. tsutsugamushi	Inoculation by bite	Scrub typhus		Infected mites Reservoir, small mammals	
R. burneti	Inhalation Ingestion	Q fever (PUO, atypical pneumonia, endocarditis)		Infected cows' milk Placenta, fetal fluids and membranes from cows and sheep	
R. mooseri	Inoculation	Endemic typhus fever		Rat fleas	

Virus	Entry Route	Disease	Exit Route	Usual Source of Infection	Accomodation
Chlamydiae	Inhalation	Psittacosis (ornithosis)	Respiratory secretions	Parrots, budgerigars and many birds. Venereal contact	Single room during acute febrile phase
	Inoculation by contact	Lymphogranuloma venereum	Discharge from lesions		
	Contact	TRIC virus (trachoma, inclusion conjunctivitis) Keratoconjunctivitis and related conditions	Discharge from lesions	Associated with overcrowding and poor sanitation in tropical countries. Fomites, flies	Single room for 48 hours tetracycline or sulphonamide then ward
		Non-specific urethritis and cervicitis	Discharge from lesions	Venereal transmission	

11 Applied Microbiology

The information contained in the preceding chapters is intended to enable the reader to understand procedures designed to prevent the transmission of infection in both hospital and community. It would be easy to assume that modern technical knowledge, drugs and facilities would outdate the problem of infection. We have come a long way from the doctrine of 'laudable pus'; methods of asepsis and hygiene are well-established and a wide range of anti-microbial agents exists to treat most infections. However, this is counterbalanced by factors such as the increasing complexity of treatment for many diseases (immuno-suppression for organ transplants; cancer chemotherapy which may leave the patient susceptible to usually harmless microbes), and the ease and speed of travel which may bring 'foreign' diseases into any country. Human nature remains such that mistakes are still made.

Main factors associated with hospital infection
● Hospitals by definition are places to which the sick are brought for treatment. In addition to those coming in for planned surgical procedures, many will be suffering from infections ranging from gastroenteritis or chest infection to diabetic ulcers and other conditions which involve the presence of pathogenic organisms. These are obviously potential sources of cross-infection within the hospital.

● All staff and patients carry organisms, some are also healthy carriers of pathogenic bacteria, others are known to be infected. The sheer numbers of people contained within a limited area favours the spread of organisms. A ward may only contain twenty patients but many more will pass through the area in a working day.

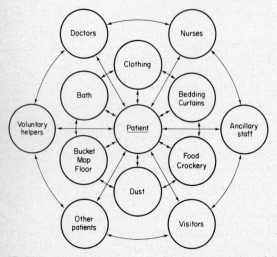

Fig. 47. The cross-infection carousel. (By kind permission of *Nursing Mirror*.)

● Antibiotics will be in use for some of those already infected. This can lead in both patients and staff to the suppression of relatively sensitive organisms in favour of highly resistant strains which can colonize an individual or a whole area.

● Special units may involve particular hazards. Renal units use dialysis machinery with potential risk to the patient from any infection and to the staff from possible hepatitis B carriers (serum hepatitis). Intensive therapy units care for severely ill patients, a proportion of whom will be artificially ventilated, fed intravenously and catheterized—all procedures that bypass the natural defences of the body.

Special care baby units involve care of those highly susceptible to infection for immunological reasons who also need frequent handling and feeding, increasing opportunities for infection transfer.

● The susceptibility of many patients to pathogenic organisms varies widely according to their general and local powers of resistance.

> *General factors* include:
>> Age: in infancy immune mechanisms may not be fully developed, and in old age at least some of these mechanisms are impaired
>> Nutritional states affect resistance
>> Immune mechanisms are interfered with by steroid drugs and cancer chemotherapy in diseases such as leukaemia, and in organ transplants
>> Diseases requiring treatment with antibiotics or ionizing radiation will also affect a patient's resistance to infection
>
> *Local factors* include:
>> Diseases such as diabetes or peripheral vascular disease involve poor blood supply and the presence of necrotic tissue. This establishes good conditions for the multiplication of certain bacteria
>> Investigations which bypass the normal defences increase the risk of introducing infection, e.g. catheterization, biopsy, radiography

We must therefore accept that infection will always be present somewhere in a hospital and aim to prevent its transmission. The nurse needs to think about the three elements vital to allowing the spread of infection:

—source of infection
—susceptible host
—means of transmission

Control and prevention will be aimed at all three but chiefly at prevention of transmission by:

Removing the source of infection either by treatment and/or isolation of the patient and by adequate disinfection and sterilization of relevant contaminated articles.

Protecting the susceptible host by immunization when necessary or applicable; screening of hospital personnel where relevant; and, in surgery, by sterilization of all objects coming in contact with the patient's tissues and with minimal handling of the latter.

Blocking the lines of communication which would permit transmission by isolation of infected or highly susceptible patients; by use of strict aseptic techniques; control of carriers; and scrupulous hygiene in all hospital areas (including food preparation, waste disposal, laundry services and housekeeping programmes).

Measures to prevent transmission of infection can be discussed under the following headings:

Architectural design and facilities
Hygiene—environmental and personal
Aseptic practice
Education
Isolation/segregation of infected patients

Architectural design and facilities
New hospitals are being built, experienced nurses are working with planning teams and many more nurses are now consulted about the detail of ward and departmental planning. The main areas of concern related to infection control are:

● Separation of clean and dirty activities such as treatment and dirty utility areas in wards, with traffic flow always leading from clean to dirty areas. This facilitates good practice, remembering that people will always be the main factor in transmitting infection.

● Adequate spacing between beds to allow correct working procedures, and the prevention of direct transmission of respiratory organisms from one patient to the next. As a working guide, bed centres should be at least 2.5 m apart and where beds are opposite each other a distance of not less than 2 m between foot-ends is recommended (Department of Health and Social Security 1968). Overcrowding increases the risk of cross-infection.

● Provisions of a high enough percentage of beds in single rooms with facilities for hand washing and storage or protective clothing in anterooms so that infected patients and those at risk from infection can be effectively segregated and safely nursed.

● Selection of surfaces and finishes is necessary so that they are not only aesthetically pleasing but can be efficiently and economically cleaned. The modern trend towards carpeting even some clinical areas has been shown by some careful scientific studies to have microbiological dangers in the accumulation of bacteria within the pile, as well as the obvious difficulty of removing hospital spills, blood, urine or chemicals. Basin and bath overflow drains should be omitted. They are impossible to keep clean and are commonly heavily contaminated with *Pseudomonas aeruginosa* and coliform organisms.

● Ventilation systems and control of airflow, designed and maintained to keep the environment as uncontaminated as possible. Stairwells, lifts and chutes as well as doors and windows have an effect on the movement and direction of airflow in a multi-storey building. Opening ward windows to produce a current of fresh air not only makes the atmosphere more pleasant but also reduces the number of organisms by diluting their concentration. In the operating theatre where tissues normally protected by the skin and other natural barriers are exposed for a considerable time, it is important for the air to be as clean as possible; air is therefore filtered, humidified, warmed or cooled, delivered and extracted at a measured rate by the air conditioning plant. The circulation and direction in which air flows is also important; theatre suites are described in 'zones': sterile, clean and dirty; the pressure being highest in the sterile preparation room and theatre and lowest in the changing and sluice rooms so that the air flows from sterile to clean to dirty zones—never in reverse.

In patient-protection units as well as in operating theatres the aims are:

To introduce pathogen-free air

To prevent contaminated air entering by other routes, e.g. doors

To minimize contamination from the environment

To remove bacteria as rapidly as possible from the vicinity of the patient

The median diameter of pathogenic bacteria-carrying particles in air is about 12 μm, range 4–24. In practice, filters with 99.9% efficiency at 5 μm pass air suitable for operating theatre suites.

Laminar air flow clean rooms have recently received publicity for their use in hospital in operating theatres, organ transplant and special care units. In a laminar airflow room, air moving at high speed (often 30 m per minute) is introduced through a filter bank which takes the place of the whole of one wall (horizontal flow), or the entire ceiling (vertical flow), and is extracted through the opposite wall in the first case and at floor level in the other. The principal advantage of laminar airflow ventilation is the rate at which the organisms are removed from the vicinity of the patient. Provided that neither person nor object moves or projects between the air source (i.e. one wall in horizontal flow or the ceiling in vertical flow) and the patient, the possibility of the transfer of organisms is minimal. This fact in no way diminishes the possibility of contact transmission by staff carrying out medical or nursing procedures, or of self-contamination by the patient.

● Design should allow for safe delivery of clean/sterile materials to the wards (CSSD, food etc.) and safe storage and removal of used instruments, waste and linen. Separate and sufficient handwashing facilities for staff and patients must be provided.

● Animals and insects can spread disease. Hospitals, particularly the kitchens, should be designed to exclude this possibility, e.g. fly screens, rat-proof stores. Pharaoh's ants have been found in sterile packs, encouraged by the warmth of central heating systems, and evidence exists of their ability to carry pathogenic bacteria. Adequate pest control programmes are needed to prevent or eradicate infestations with these and other pests.

The nurse on the ward has a role in maintaining safe use of these facilities: reporting breakdowns in equipment, failure of supplies and observing the rules for care of patients nursed in isolation.

Hygiene—environmental and personal

Basic personal hygiene, such as hand-washing (probably the most important measure in prevention of cross-infection) must be observed after all procedures involving bed-making, pressure area care, temperature-taking, removal of excreta, any service to patients in isolation and before and after any aseptic procedures. Wet hands provide an excellent media for many micro-organisms to thrive and be transferred—thorough drying and safe disposal of the towel will eliminate many of these. Communal articles such as cakes of soap and roller towels should be discouraged; pots of hand cream should be banned and individual tubes substituted.

Personal hygiene will include clean nails, hair and uni-form—all potential conveyors of infection. Protective gowns or aprons will be used for certain activities including aseptic procedures and nursing patients in isolation.

Staff should be aware that prompt reporting of diarrhoea, sore throats, purulent discharges, boils, styes, whitlows and septic cuts or burns is in the interest of patients as well as themselves.

Environmental hygiene includes the physical removal of dust and dirt from wards and corridors. Methods of clean-ing designed with regard to control of infection include the use of vacuum cleaners with filtered air exhausts, scrubbing machines, safe containment and disposal of waste materials to incineration and of dirty linen to the laundry. Nurses can help by organizing activities with domestic staff to avoid, for example, dressings coinciding with ward cleaning.

Hygiene in kitchens is vital—food, water, milk and ice may all be causes of food poisoning, e.g. due to staphylo-coccal enterotoxin, *Clostridium welchii, Salmonella* or *Shigella,* or diseases such as typhoid fever, tuberculosis or brucellosis. The staff and all patients are susceptible; babies under a year old are at particularly high risk because they lack one of the natural defence barriers to intestinal infection—stomach hydrochloric acid.

Patients receiving extensive antibiotic therapy, those with low white blood cell counts and babies are also very susceptible to mouth infection caused by *Candida* sp. (*Monilia,* thrush) which is easily spread from patient to patient by inadequately processed feeding equipment and crockery, e.g. cups, bottle teats, medicine spoons and glasses. Other organisms such as *Streptococcus pyogenes* or tubercle bacilli may be transferred in this way; the bacteria being protected in inaccessible cracks or in dried sputum or saliva. There is no place for perfunctory washing-up procedures and the use of cracked or chipped crockery should be prevented. If a washing-up machine with liberal supplies of very hot water is not available, it is necessary to boil utensils after use by a patient with any mouth or throat infection.

In this country there are statutory regulations concerning food supplies. Certain standards are required in restaurants and institutions; these relate to kitchen hygiene, the storage and handling of food, staff health, conditions of work and personal hygiene, e.g. the provision of clean uniform, hand-washing and toilet facilities.

Communal items are always bacteriologically suspect. A critical appraisal of equipment is needed to arrange appropriate cleaning and decontamination of anything used communally or by a succession of patients, to prevent the spread of infection by indirect contact. For example:

Mouth and respiratory tract infections, e.g. *Streptococcus pyogenes* or *Candida* sp., may be transmitted by nursing equipment such as thermometers, inhalation or oral hygiene equipment as well as by incubators, respirators and humidifiers. *Staphylococcus aureus* is easily transferred from skin to talcum powder used for pressure area care.

Communal towels, wheelchair blankets, bath mats, soft toys, or pillows not enclosed in plastic cases, all show bacteriological evidence of their recent users and may be responsible for an outbreak of cross-infection. Nevertheless, hygiene in terms of hand-washing remains the single most important measure the nurse can take to help prevent spread of infection.

Aseptic techniques

The principle of asepsis is to prevent the introduction of micro-organisms into sites that are normally free of them, or in normally non-sterile areas to avoid the introduction of micro-organisms from outside sources. This covers a wide range of activities from the operating department, where all materials that can come into contact with tissues are sterilized, to a radiographer or physiotherapist replacing a dressing, a physician aspirating a chest, a medical student or house officer passing a catheter, an anaesthetist giving a spinal anaesthetic, and a nurse removing sutures or aspirating a tracheostomy. The following principles and requirements apply:

1. A clean environment and adequate working space (already discussed).

2. *Sterile supplies,* including dressings, instruments, lotions and equipment. Sterile supplies used in a hospital come from various sources; they may be commercially prepacked and sterilized, supplied by a local or regional Central Sterile Supply Department (CSSD), by the pharmacy, or processed in a department such as an operating theatre. While it is usually the responsibility of the bacteriologist and the Control of Infection Committee to advise on methods of sterilization, packaging, and safe storage and the responsibility of the Nursing Procedure Committee to advise on selection, opening and procedure, it is the responsibility of every user to check that each pack is undamaged before use and opened in the prescribed manner so that the sterility of the content is preserved.

Sterilizing methods are discussed in Chapter 7 and *indicators* in Appendix I. The outer container should be labelled with the method and date of processing, and an appropriate sterilizing indicator. The *packing and presentation of sterile supplies* is subject to central as well as local control. Many pharmaceutical preparations are manufactured to exacting requirements; expert committees convened by the Department of Health and Social Security study and recommend standards for packaging materials and methods of packing.

Packaging materials should facilitate sterilization, for example, allow steam penetration, but also act as a barrier to insects, dust or moisture which could carry bacteria into the pack. Incorrect packing or wrapping will invalidate the sterilizing procedure. For example, nylon film is steam permeable but the time taken to evacuate air from the pack and achieve steam penetration is far in excess of the normal autoclave cycle time, making this an unsuitable wrap for this sterilization method. Substandard paper bags or inadequately heat-sealed plastic or paper, or poor fold closures will allow pack content contamination after sterilization.

In considering the *storage of sterile supplies* the aim is to preserve sterility not to challenge it with severe tests. It is therefore recommended that:

a. Supplies are stored well off the floor, in a clean, dry area.

b. In an even temperature.

c. Protected from dust. Any accumulated dust will be disseminated at the time of opening and is likely to settle on the sterile field.

d. Shelf and container surfaces should be smooth for ease of cleaning and to prevent damage to the packs.

e. Supplies should be used in strict rotation to avoid deterioration.

f. 'Shelf life' (prescribed storage time) will depend to some extent on local conditions. It is generally agreed that paper-wrapped packs present the problem. Waterproof plastic and metal can be swabbed with a suitable antiseptic to remove accumulated dust, which in a hospital is likely to contain pathogens. Given intact and efficient wraps, it is probable that sterilized pack contents remain sterile for a long time but in the case of paper-wrapped packs (where damp swabbing to remove dust would certainly contaminate the content) it is impossible to open the pack without contaminating the content with the dust which has collected on the outer wrap. Double wraps are considered to be safe than a single layer because the inner wrap acts as a barrier to dust and bacteria disturbed when the outer layer is opened. The longer a pack is stored, the more dust accumulates on the outside, and the greater the chance of contamination on opening. For this reason turnover should be as fast as possible to ensure the shortest practicable shelf life.

Many pharmaceutical preparations are marked with an expiry date after which they should not be used, others have a colour indicator incorporated which changes when the chemical loses its activity.

It is easy and wrong to assume that all lotions, ointments, creams and antiseptics in the ward cupboards are sterile. Fluids, including antiseptics, are very easily contaminated by contact with a hand, a swab or a dropped and replaced stopper. An antiseptic may be effective against one group of bacteria but totally ineffective against another group, e.g. cetrimide is active against staphylococci but will allow *Pseudomonas aeruginosa* to survive; staphylococci unlike most other organisms can survive in saline. A Winchester of distilled water used to 'top-up' humidifiers, although sterile when issued, may easily become contaminated by a wet medium organism such as *Klebsiella* sp. which will then multiply, infect the humidifier at the next filling, and then the patient. Hand cream by the ward basin, contaminated by an unwashed hand may pass a pathogenic organism on to the next user who washes before carrying out a clean procedure for a patient. Patients should be supplied with individual containers of creams or ointments, particularly when they are to be applied to the skin by hand. Recommendations in 1969 (HM(69)86 *Preservation of sterility in ophthalmic preparations used in hospitals*), concerning eye medications emphasize the serious risk of cross-infection where communal stock containers of eye drops or ointments are used. Each patient should have his own drops or ointments applied with a sterilized pipette or rod, or single dose applicators should be used. See also Chapter 7.

3. *Skin and hair* are never sterile. In addition to the normal skin flora, both pick up and transiently carry any organism with which they are in contact. This is one reason for the preoperative shaving of a patient's body hair, and for covering the hair of staff working in operating theatres and certain high-risk areas. Both the skin of the patients and the hands of the operator are thoroughly washed and dried to remove transient contaminating bacteria, particular attention being paid to skin creases, e.g. between the fingers, the umbilicus, etc. To remove any remaining surface bacteria an antiseptic, e.g. iodine, chlorhexidine, is applied to the operation area before the skin is incised or punctured.

4. The use of *protective clothing* and *non-touch technique* to prevent organisms from the operator reaching vulnerable patient tissues:

Gowns. Skin particles and bacteria are constantly shed, the clothing and shoes of a normal individual carry these and other micro-organisms picked up by contact with people and objects. Although there is doubt as to the risk from many of these micro-organisms, some contact transference of potential pathogens is inevitable and would almost certainly result in cross-infection and so a clean gown (sterile in certain situations) is worn when carrying out aseptic procedures.

Closely woven fabric is a barrier to bacteria when dry but allows them to pass in both directions when wet. If a surgeon gets his sterile gown wet with blood or saline, bacteria from the patient will be in contact with his skin. Conversely, bacteria from the surgeon's skin and the clothing under his gown will gain access to the wound. It is most important for all members of the staff to change into fresh theatre clothing and shoes before entering the clean zone of the operating theatre or other areas where patients are at high risk from infection (as with burns or protective isolation) and every effort is made to keep the numbers of micro-organisms to a minimum. Disposable plastic gowns or aprons are in use in many hospitals for dressings and for nursing patients in other categories of isolation.

Gloves. To avoid direct contact between the skin of the operator and the patient, either non-touch technique, i.e. forceps instead of fingers are used, or sterile gloves are worn. Dressings and sterile equipment are handled by the same means to avoid indirect transmission of organisms.

Masks. 'Deflector' masks, designed to deflect expired air away from the immediate area (thus preventing wound contamination), e.g. simple paper masks.
'Filter' masks, designed to protect the wearer from inhalation of airborne organisms by trapping them in the mask fibres, e.g. close-fitting glass fibre type.
Both types are effective only when dry. When masks are worn they should be discarded when not required; handling a used mask, storing it in a pocket or wearing it intermitently dropped around the neck are serious infection risks. Use of 'deflector' masks for ward dressings and other procedures is a matter for individual hospital policies; they are essential to theatre work and the nursing care of patients with burns and high-risk patients.

Caps. Hair should always be restrained since it disperses bacteria freely when moving. It should be completely covered by a cap when this constitutes a risk to the patient, e.g. for protective isolation, and in the operating theatre.

5. Clean procedures should always be carried out before those known or suspected to be infected.

6. When opening ward procedure packs:

a. Check that the pack is undamaged.

b. Check that the pack has been through a sterilizing process (indicator).

c. Check that prescribed storage time (if relevant) has not been exceeded.

d. If the bags are not designed to peel or unfold, cut with clean scissors reserved for the purpose. Tearing paper disperses fragments and dust from the surface.

e. The *inner wrapper* of the pack is opened to form the sterile field by handling the corners of the wrapper only, opening away from the body so that it is never necessary to reach across the *sterile field*.

f. Only sterile materials are placed on the sterile field; these and the field itself are only touched by sterile forceps or sterile gloved hands. Once sterile swabs have been in contact with the patient's wound and skin they are no longer sterile, therefore they are never replaced on the sterile field or redipped into sterile lotion but discarded and a new swab taken.

7. An important aspect of infection control is the *safe disposal* of all used material. Used dressings and instruments should be contained at the point of use, in suitable wet-strength bags for transportation to the incinerator and service departments.

Isolation/segregation of infected patients

The most obvious way to block the lines of communication which allow transmission of infection, is to physically segregate any patient with a known or suspected infection. The extent of this isolation will depend on the organism's mode of spread—precautions taken to prevent spread by airborne routes are obviously different to those for direct contact. There are two main methods of isolation:

> *Source isolation*—to contain infection and prevent its transmission ('barrier nursing').
> *Protective isolation*—where the patient is at risk from infection and needs protection from all possible micro-organisms ('reverse barrier nursing').

Patients may be nursed in the following types of isolation accommodation:

1. Specially designated hospitals for the care of patients suffering from or suspected of having one of a few specific diseases—currently smallpox, Lassa fever, Marburg disease and other viral haemorrhagic fevers. This may be either within an infectious diseases hospital temporarily used for care of these cases only, or in a hospital reserved for and independently staffed for the care (at this time) of smallpox cases or suspects only.

2. Isolation units/infectious diseases hospitals—these may either be attached to a general hospital or separate entities. In 1971 the Department of Health and Social Security suggested that each district general hospital should have an isolation unit for the care of all infectious diseases except those in category 1.

3. Single rooms attached to general wards—where the majority of isolation takes place in older hospitals. Staff and facilities are shared with the rest of the ward, but this

should be quite adequate for both contact and airborne infections if nursing techniques are properly applied. Ideally there should be an anteroom for changing and hand-washing facilities for staff, and separate toilet and wash facilities for the patient.

4. 'Barrier nursing' in a general ward—suitable for some infections spread by contact routes, e.g. hepatitis A and salmonella infections (if the patient is continent and not confused). This is of no value in airborne infections, and scrupulous techniques must be adhered to by all staff if this is to be effective 'isolation'. The clinical state of infection, in addition to the causative organism, must be considered—a wound that is heavily discharging is a hazard whatever the cause and will probably require care in a single room.

5. Protective isolation units—whether portable 'plastic tent isolators' or more permanent structures. They are in use in some hospitals for high-risk patients whose immune mechanisms are compromised. The tents permit good access to the patient and reduce the sense of 'isolation' caused by single room separation.

All personnel need to understand the procedures involved in caring for individuals nursed in isolation, and the patient must be helped to see that it is his disease which is being isolated and not himself. (Both these points will be considered in detail in the following chapter). As his most frequent contact the nurse is in the best position to reassure the patient.

Staff need policies to follow in order that infected patients are admitted into appropriate accommodation. These policies need to be kept under review and the control of infection officer or his deputy (see page 211) should always be available for advice.

Education

Nursing, medical and paramedical staff need thorough appreciation of the need for asepsis and hygienic procedures; domestic and catering staff need to understand the hygienic precautions taken in their areas of work and so on. Only then will unnecessary infection be prevented.

It is unfortunate that the link between a break in technique and the appearance of hospital-acquired infection is often hard to demonstrate, and that a certain level of infection is virtually accepted as 'normal' by many people; others manage to ignore the very existence of infection. Staff should all be encouraged to feel a personal responsibility in preventing and controlling hospital infection. Studies have shown that infection rates are reduced when it is known that procedures are being monitored.

Occupational health departments can be of great help in promoting standards. They see and assess staff on employment, talk to various groups of employees and liaise with the microbiology department concerning sick staff. They can explain to staff attending their department with skin or gastro-intestinal infections, influenza or streptococcal sore throats that they are a hazard to others and arrange appropriate moves. The Infection Control Nurse (see page 211) can help a great deal by being 'on-the-spot' to try and increase staff awareness of infection risks and to observe how well policies are being adhered to.

CONTROL OF INFECTION TEAM

Despite provision of well-designed hospitals, well-taught staff, satisfactory policies of hygiene, sterilization and disinfection, asepsis and appropriate isolation of infected patients, it is still possible for cross-infection to occur if there are no specified personnel to ensure that policies are taught, applied and coordinated. The responsibility for implementation of these policies and their supervision rests with Area Health Authorities who initiate the formation of a Control of Infection Committee and appointment of a Control of Infection Officer. Committee membership will vary between hospitals, partly depending on their size and function, but may include membership from all main departments: medical, nursing, administration, occupational health, community physician, engineering, domestic, pharmacy, CSSD and microbiology. Close links with the community are helpful for standardization of policies throughout the district.

Responsibilities of the control of infection committee
1. Concern with the numbers of nosocomial infections brought to them by the control of infection officer.
2. Introducing, modifying and maintaining policies on:
    Isolation
    Admission of infected patients
    Aseptic techniques and practice
    Standardization of supplies, etc
    Antibiotic management
3. Liaising with the Occupational Health Department.
4. Involvement in in-service training programmes.
5. Ensuring that adequate microbiological facilities exist.

The control of infection officer. This post is often held by a microbiologist. He is responsible for awareness of the incidence of infection within the hospital in order to recognize any change in the 'normal' pattern, to investigate and if possible prevent any spread of infection. He must be empowered to act when necessary without having to convene the committee, and should be available to offer advice on matters of infection control, hygiene, disinfection and so on. As he usually has a full-time appointment already, many hospitals appoint an assistant, generally a nurse.

Infection control nurse. This post is best held by a nurse rather than by a microbiology technician, a doctor, or any other individual with apparently useful specialist knowledge, as nurses are trained in patient-handling procedures and so can assess how these are being performed. The nurse will, of course, need extra knowledge of microbiology, laboratory techniques and tests, and a broad view of management problems in order to achieve useful co-operation with all hospital departments.

The nurse is usually responsible to the District Nursing Officer but technically responsible to the Control of Infection Officer and acts under his guidance. He may be at charge nurse or nursing officer level—according to the size of the post and to previous experience. Ideally he will be able to enter all hospital areas and communicate freely with all levels of staff in order to assess the efficiency of hospital policies and seek early evidence of their breakdown or infection. The post requires tact and firmness in dealing with a variety of people, obtaining required information and motivating personnel to implement infection control policies. The precise role of an ICN in Great Britain will vary according to the size and nature of the hospitals and the way the post is seen by district or divisional nursing officer and microbiologist (if there is a microbiologist for the nurse to work with). The following gives an outline of one post:

Role of infection control nurse

To help achieve and maintain the highest possible standards of practice, with particular regard to the safety of patients and staff against all hazards of infection, in conjunction with the infection control team. Duties will fall into the following broad categories:

Advice and liaison. To advise on matters relating to infection, hospital hygiene, techniques of sterilization and disinfection, and care of patients requiring isolation.

Teaching. Formally and informally to all grades of nursing, professional and ancillary staff. This includes lectures to student and pupil nurses and participation in in-service training to many grades of staff. A great deal is taught on informal visits around the hospital: explaining the reasons for certain procedures, answering queries and offering advice. This extends to all hospital personnel.

Monitoring and research. This involves awareness of the state of infection in the hospital day by day, following up situations as necessary from scrutiny of ward and laboratory reports, involving frequent visits to both areas. This is an ideal time for offering advice, helping enforce hospital isolation policies, promptly identifying infected patients and reporting any difficulties experienced.

In addition to this daily activity, anything unusual and all outbreaks of infection will be investigated and reports kept for the Control of Infection Officer and Committee. New equipment and supplies will involve the ICN and Supplies and other departments in possible trials. Procedure committees will be part of the ICN's role and to keep abreast of technical advances they will need to read relevant medical and nursing journals. Contact with fellow workers is also important and membership of the Infection Control Nurses Association and other bodies will be encouraged.

The ICN needs to establish and maintain a good relationship with all grades and divisions of hospital personnel, including:

Nursing staff, students, pupils, tutors, administration staff.
Medical staff and students.
Department heads in CSSD, supplies, laundry, catering, domestic management, pharmacy, engineering, hospital administration, physiotherapy, voluntary workers, etc. and their employees.
Technicians and staff of the pathology department.

In cases of staff sickness the ICN may become aware of a sudden increase in sore throats, diarrhoea and vomiting, etc. and can alert the Occupational Health Department, encouraging affected staff to attend. The nurse may also inform the OHD of the distribution of patients who represent a specific hazard such as cases of active pulmonary tuberculosis, so that staff immunity may be checked where necessary.

Occupational health departments

As already mentioned, the staff of these departments are closely involved with hospital infection control programmes. They should ideally be responsible for the health and safety of all personnel employed in the hospital or community. In addition to health interviews and medical assessment before or upon employment, they will check immunization status regarding tuberculosis, poliomyelitis (and rubella in the cases of female staff of child-bearing age). In susceptible cases they will offer the necessary vaccination or immunization.

They may check that staff are fit to return to work after illness or infections including boils, as well as other minor sepsis, e.g. gastro-intestinal or streptococcal infections. They work with the Control Infection Officer and nurse to formulate policies for special hazards in order to avoid staff infection, and maintain records on all staff infection. Their role in the education of many groups of staff with regard to prevention has already been mentioned.

The community nursing services and infection control

Nurses from hospitals are increasingly involved with community 'modules', and infected patients go home sooner to be cared for by community staff. Health visitors and midwives are involved with mothers and babies sent home 48 h after delivery, and patients admitted or discharged with pulmonary tuberculosis and other diseases have families in need of advice and reassurance. Staff involved in their care must be kept informed of the details of each individual's condition to help protect both the patient and all contacts.

Community health centres and general practitioner surgeries face problems similar to hospitals in terms of design, amenities and disposal of infected materials, if on a different scale. Many hospital policies can and should be modified for use in the community according to the resources available; these may range from care of patients infested with scabies or lice (increasing in many urban areas), to safe disposal of needles, syringes and soiled dressings. Sterile, single-use supplies are increasingly available to staff in the community as well as the hospital, and the same protective methods should also be available to them. These include single-use plastic aprons, and unsterile disposable gloves to prevent gross contamination during some procedures. Disinfectant and other solutions including medications are all potential sources of infection and a system of safe storage and supply needs arrangement. The development of alcoholic hand-washing preparations such as Hibisol should help community nurses in that most basic aid to controlling infection—careful hand-washing.

Community nurses can also play a major part in controlling infection by health education. They can teach both patient and relatives about care in disposal of dressings, sensible hygiene with regard to hand-washing, care of indwelling catheters and similar concerns. At all times they will have to exercise great tact to maintain good relationships whilst successfully advising patients and their families.

12 Isolation Techniques

The need to prevent transmission of infection from one individual to another is by now apparent. A brief description of how isolation techniques play their part was given in the previous chapter. The aim of the next two chapters is to describe in some detail the actual methods which can be used and to discuss the problems which these can cause— and how the nurse can play a major part in alleviating them.

The history of isolating infected patients to prevent their being the cause of further infection goes back hundreds of years and has been fraught with misconceptions, unwarranted fears and prejudices. This has caused much unnecessary suffering to the truly 'isolated' person. Many of these mistaken ideas arose before the epidemiology of diseases was understood, before antimicrobial drugs existed to treat infections, and before there was any detailed understanding of immunity. Once drugs and vaccines to treat and protect people were discovered, and the routes for spread of diseases became understood, logical procedures to prevent transmission could be developed and applied. It is regrettable to note that this often failed to happen and even today there is a tendency for people to react with a degree of panic to many infections. This causes the sufferer to be far more 'isolated' than his disease requires. Conversely a cavalier attitude may be taken that 'there is no real problem' of cross-infection. Both need eradicating through education.

New trends

In the 1970s new developments have made it vital to understand how each disease is transmitted in order to contain it with the maximum safety and minimum effort. These include:

1. The speed of jet travel with increased risk of importing 'exotic' diseases such as Lassa fever from Africa to Europe.

2. The closing of many infectious disease ('fever') hospitals and their replacement by isolation units in general hospitals, (and the use of single rooms attached to general wards), for containment of quite severe infections.

3. The increased use and range of antimicrobial drugs which has also meant an increase in hospital-acquired strains of antibiotic resistant pathogens.

4. A new class of patient needing protection from the environment due to immunosuppression (e.g. transplant patients), immune deficiency or drug-induced vulnerability (e.g. treatment of some leukaemias).

PRINCIPLES OF NURSING CARE OF INFECTED PATIENTS

When a patient presents with an infection, any action taken should be designed to prevent the transmission of pathogenic micro-organisms directly or indirectly, via airborne particles, fluids, equipment or food to other patients, staff or visitors. Many hospitals have only a limited number of single rooms which have to be allocated to the best advantage of all patients and it is important that the patients selected for these rooms are truly in need of them. Misuse of the facilities will lead to wasted time and expense and accompanying disillusion. These questions will identify how to deal with each infection and must be asked:

1. What is the causative organism?
2. Where is it?
3. By which route does it leave the body?
4. Are other patients or staff vulnerable?
5. Is segregation essential, advisable or unnecessary?

With the answers provided, appropriate precautions can be taken and understood by both patient and staff.

General principles
● The environment is kept clean and well ventilated to reduce the number of micro-organisms. Equipment is kept to a minimum.
● Always wash and dry hands after contact with an infected person or his bedding, personal effects or excreta. Hands are the commonest agents in transmission of infection.

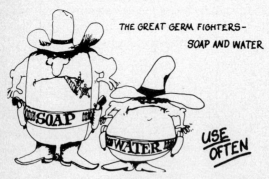

THE GREAT GERM FIGHTERS—
SOAP AND WATER

USE OFTEN

● Limit the number of people in direct contact with an infected person, and check their state of immunity where possible.
● Safely contain all infected material at the point of use— including all dressings, tissues, bedding and other secretion-soiled items. Dispatch for incineration or disinfection/sterilization in appropriate containers, secure and distinguishable. 'Double-bagging' may be used. This

means placing contaminated articles into appropriate bags in the patient's room and transferring them into an outer container at the exit from the room.

Methods
Hospitals require specific policies to follow when caring for infected patients. Many are now using systems which attempt to prevent transmission of infection by assigning patients to one of a number of isolation categories according to the nature and severity of the disease and its route of spread. These categories have appropriate techniques assigned to them (see below). Alternatively, a policy may be made which alphabetically lists all infections likely to be encountered and describes the specific precautions to be taken for each and every infection or disease. Each hospital will have to decide which is the best system for it to use and the method will be more likely to succeed if all departments are consulted before its institution.

If an alphabetical list is used, the following headings will allow a guideline to be developed:

Infection—Reservoir of infecting agent—Entry route—Exit route—Isolation—Gown—Mask—Gloves—Containment of infected linen—Disinfection of equipment—Terminal disinfection—Availability of artificially acquired immunity—Incubation period. The necessity for isolation follows on the details of the routes of transmission and the need for particular protective measures can then be filled in. This system attempts to make staff consider the reasons behind isolation for each individual.

Categories of isolation
The following are based on the US Department of Health, Welfare and Education guidelines, but other variations exist.

'Source' isolation (see Chapter 11).
   Strict isolation
   Respiratory isolation
   Enteric isolation
   Wound and skin precautions
'Protective' isolation.

Each category contains a list of all the diseases which are appropriate to it and has a card showing what precautions are needed when caring for the affected patients. This may take the form of a printed list or a pictorial instruction, the latter being one way of overcoming the language barrier. This is attached to the door of the patient's room and should always request visitors to report to the Sister's office so that the reason for isolation and its consequent precautions can be explained. The categories will now be demonstrated but it must be stressed that these are only suggested examples and each hospital will make its own policy.

SOURCE ISOLATION

Strict isolation is for those infections that can spread by both contact and airborne routes and are highly transmissible. Some will require isolation in totally separate buildings (see Chapter 11) such as smallpox, Lassa fever, Marburg virus disease and Ebola or other viral haemorrhagic fevers. However, a few other infections will require extensive isolation techniques because of the hazard to other patients or staff, including:

   Anthrax (pulmonary or systemic)
   Burns, major, infected with *Staph. aureus* or *beta haemolytic streptococcus* Group A
   Congenital rubella syndrome
   Diphtheria
   Herpes zoster—disseminated

Plague (pneumonic)

Rabies (potential inoculation of saliva, or spitting in staff's eyes, in advanced cases)

Skin infection, major, infected with *Staph. aureus* or *beta haemolytic streptococcus* Group A

Vaccinia—generalized and eczema vaccinatum

In view of both main routes of transmission being involved, the patient will need a single room, and staff and visitors will require gowns, masks and gloves. All articles leaving the room must be safely contained prior to sending for incineration, disinfection or sterilization as appropriate and the use of disposable items is possible when convenient. Strict hand-washing must be maintained. The following is an example of a typical card for this category:

Strict Isolation

Visitors—Please Report to Sister's Office Before Entering

Single room: necessary. Door to be kept closed

Gowns/plastic aprons: must be worn by anyone entering room

Masks: must be worn by anyone entering room. 'Filter' type

Hands: must be washed on entering and leaving

Gloves: must be worn

Articles: to be safely contained for sterilization, disinfection or incineration

Before

After

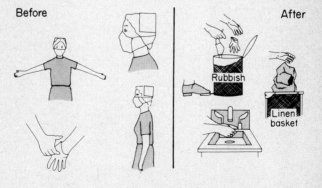

Rubbish

Linen basket

Respiratory isolation is for those infections that may be spread by direct contact or droplets, or airborne droplet nuclei in the case of tuberculosis. They are initially nursed with many of the precautions for strict isolation. The period of use of masks and gowns will depend on susceptibility of the infecting organisms to antibiotics, the length of the infective period and the immunization state of staff and visitors. It is a great help to patients if their attendants are immune and do not have to be hidden behind a mask. The diseases in this category will include the 'childhood diseases' which may still affect adults, and a few others:

> Measles
> Mumps
> Pertussis (whooping cough)
> Rubella (German measles)
> Tuberculosis (pulmonary)

Respiratory Isolation

Visitors—Please Report to Sister's Office Before Entering

Single room: necessary. Door to be kept closed

Gowns/plastic aprons: must be worn for contact with patient

Masks: must be worn unless immune. 'Filter' type

Hands: must be washed on entering and leaving

Gloves: not necessary

Articles: to be safely contained for sterilization, disinfection or incineration

Before   After

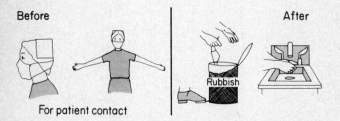

For patient contact

Rubbish

Enteric isolation is for those diseases spread by the 'faecal–oral' route through direct or indirect contact with excreta or articles faecally contaminated, involving ingestion of the pathogen. This is an area requiring particular application of common sense; in the past many patients were over isolated for enteric infections and there may still be a tendency to do this. If the patient is adult, continent and has good personal hygiene, very few enteric infections require isolation in a single room—nor do attendant staff require masks! Infants, children, the incontinent and confused will, however, need a single-room. The diseases in this category can include:

> Amoebic dysentery
> Cholera
> Gastroenteritis:
> > undiagnosed, suspected infectious origin, entero-pathogenic *E. coli*
> > *Salmonella* species
> > *Shigella* species
> > *Yersinia enterocolitis*
> Hepatitis A, some types of non-A, non-B hepatitis
> Poliomyelitis
> Typhoid fever (*Salmonella typhi*)

Enteric Isolation

Visitors—Please Report to Sister's Office Before Entering

Single room: for paediatric, incontinent or confused patients only

Gowns/plastic aprons: must be worn for contact with patient

Masks: not required

Hands: must be washed after contact with patient and on leaving

Gloves: must be worn for contact with patient or faecally contaminated articles

Articles: disinfection or incineration of urine or faecally contaminated articles

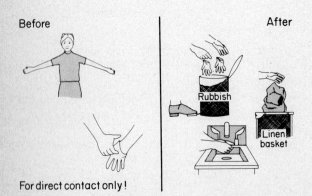

Before

After

For direct contact only!

Wound and skin precautions are designed to prevent transmission of infection by direct contact with discharging or draining wound or skin lesions and heavily contaminated articles. If the organism concerned is also a danger in respiratory spread, is highly resistant to antibiotic therapy, or the wound or lesion is discharging copiously, then a single room will be necessary. Isolation facilities are at a premium in most hospitals, however, and the need for isolation must be individually and carefully assessed if mutual cooperation is to be maintained. Medical and nursing staff should have the necessary guidelines, the infection control nurse and control of infection officer should be available to give advice, with authority to order isolation until they can discuss the case with the clinician. The following are likely to be included:

Extensive burns not in strict isolation
Gas gangrene
Herpes zoster—localized
Puerperal sepsis
Wound and skin infections not requiring strict isolation but heavily discharging or antibiotic resistant.

Wound and Skin Precautions

Visitors—Please Report to Sister's Office Before Entering

Single room: desirable

Gowns/plastic aprons: must be worn for contact with patient

Masks: only during dressing changes

Hands: must be washed after contact with patient, on entering and leaving room

Gloves: must be worn for contact with infected area and contaminated articles

Articles: linen, dressings and instruments must be safely identified and contained prior to disinfection, sterilization or incineration

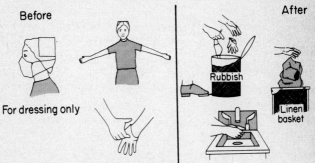

Before

For dressing only

For direct contact only!

After

Rubbish

Linen basket

'PROTECTIVE' ISOLATION ('REVERSE BARRIER NURSING')

This is designed to prevent the acquisition of infection by persons with impaired resistance or increased susceptibility to pathogens or potential pathogens in the hospital environment. It is important that medical and nursing staff attending these patients are free from transmissible infection. The measures taken will depend on the level of risk involved, and the conditions requiring this form of isolation will be a matter for individual clinical consideration. Those with mildly impaired immunity may require only a single room and the wearing of protective clothing by attendant staff. Patients suffering immunosuppression or loss of natural protective mechanisms due to disease and/or treatment, e.g. leukaemia, lymphoma, may require all articles coming into patient contact to be sterilized or disinfected, including food and drink. This also involves need for considerable psychological support for the patient. Guidelines can only be general, each occasion requiring individual consideration, but may include:

Agranulocytosis
Dermatitis or eczematous disease if severe and extensive
Non-infected severe burns
Lymphomas and leukaemias in certain instances.

Protective Isolation

Visitors—Please Report to Sister's Office Before Entering

Single room: necessary. Door to be kept closed

Gowns/plastic aprons: must be worn by anyone entering room

Masks: must be worn by anyone entering room. 'Filter' type

Hands: must be washed on entering and for procedures

Gloves: for direct contact and aseptic procedures

Articles: according to degree of protection they may be disinfected or
sterilized before entry

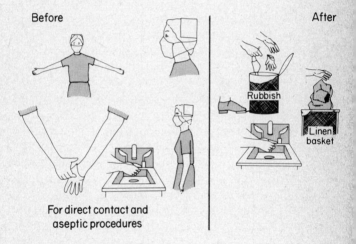

Before

After

Rubbish

Linen basket

For direct contact and
aseptic procedures

Hepatitis B (serum hepatitis)

This is worth mentioning in some detail as it is potentially a considerable problem in terms of hospital cross-infection. The virus is chiefly transmitted via the blood and, almost inevitably in hospital, venepuncture or greater surgical interference will take place. (Faeces, urine, saliva could be important in hospital spread only when contaminated with blood). The other problem is that apart from obviously jaundiced patients who should be recognized as a hazard on admission, a proportion of the population will be carrying hepatitis B surface antigen (Hb_sAg/Australia antigen) in their serum. These people may well have no clinical symptoms to alert staff to the potential danger.

Each hospital will ideally have a policy for hepatitis B patients. A list of individuals having a higher likelihood of carrying HB_sAg in their serum (including all jaundiced patients, all those with liver disease, those who have received haemodialysis or multiple transfusions, drug addicts, promiscuous homosexuals and those from countries with a high prevalence), should be circulated in order that the patient falling into these categories may be tested as soon as possible. There are a variety of tests for the presence of HB_sAg, the most commonly used being reversed passive haemagglutination and radioimmuno-assay.

The policy should have advice on safe venepuncture, transport of specimens to the laboratory and on laboratory methods. Many hospitals have adopted a yellow warning mark for all forms and samples from patients who may have the disease and all potentially contaminated articles. This is no substitute for sensible handling of specimens. Advice should be included for staff caring directly for the patient, and action to be taken in the event of accidental inoculation with a patient's blood. Specific high-titre anti-HB_sAg immunoglobulin may be deemed necessary.

Blood precautions are the most important but if the patient is bleeding, incontinent or acutely ill with the disease, then a single room is needed and all contact precautions must be observed. This applies if the patient also has surgery or an intravenous procedure. If the patient does need isolation then gloves and gowns should be worn for venepuncture, during dressings and when removing excreta. Extreme care is needed while disposing of needles and syringes. The former should be placed in puncture proof containers and the latter 'double-bagged' before incineration. All blood-stained articles need incineration, so disposable items are preferable. It is important that all staff achieve a balance, taking all necessary precautions but avoiding inducing a feeling of leper-like isolation for the patient.

In conclusion, the main considerations when devising policies for isolation are to keep them simple, logical and relevant and to monitor them regularly to ensure that they are being kept and do not need adjustment.

Comparative Notes on Isolation Techniques in a Single Bed Sideward

	To Segregate for Infection	*To Segregate for Patient Protection*
Aim	The patient has an infection Anything coming out of the room must be disinfected or safely contained for disposal	The patient is particularly vulnerable, requires protection from infection. Anything going into the room should be free from organisms capable of causing infection
Visitors	Exclude other patients if need be Instruct family	Essential staff and selected visitors only, to reduce the risk of contact transmission
Door	Closed Label 'Source Isolation'	Closed Label 'Protective Isolation'
Hand washing	On leaving (and for procedures)	On entering (and for procedures)
Gown	To protect staff clothing	To protect the patient from staff clothing
	Store clean supply outside room	Store clean supply outside room
	Discard inside room, contain in appropriate bag	Discard outside room in appropriate bag
Mask	Only if spread of infection is airborne. In 'high-risk' situations use 'filter' type Store outside room Discard inside room	Always 'Filter' type Put on before entry Discard outside room

Comparative Notes on Isolation Techniques in a Single Bed Sideward
(contd.)

Cap	No	According to degree of protection. If worn must completely cover the hair
Gloves	Certain instances only Disposable, polythene, single-use Sterile·or not according to purpose For serum hepatitis if handling blood or blood-contaminated excreta/secretions For intestinal infections when the patient is incontinent For heavily discharging lesions	Sterile gloves for aseptic procedures, e.g. intravenous infusion
Crockery etc.	Disposable items preferable Efficiently functioning washing-up machine (80°C or more) Condiments, sugar kept in room	Process utensils through the washing up machine immediately before serving meal *or* Sterilize (according to degree of protection)
Food	Normal Incinerate any waste	May be sterilized (according to degree of protection) Serve before other patients Select foods which have not been handled after cooking AVOID uncooked food, e.g. salads
Amenities	Paperback books. Incinerate. Toys, etc. should be disposable or of material which can be sterilized after use	Autoclave or disinfect, as appropriate, all items, e.g. books, clothing, toys

Comparative Notes on Isolation Techniques in a Single Bed Sideward
(contd.)

Furniture and equipment	Minimum	Same
	Select smooth, intact surfaces for ease of cleaning	Same
	Blinds preferable to curtains	Blinds or curtains outside room
	Individual medicines, lotions and ointments, sphygmomanometers, etc.	Same
Bed and personal linen	Clean daily	May be autoclaved
	Mattresses and pillows should be covered with impervious plastic	
	Dispose in appropriate bags, 'double-bagged' as necessary	Normal disposal outside room
Dressings, tissues	Disposes as for all such items 'Double-bag' for incineration	Normal disposal, outside room
Needles, syringes	Should be disposable	Same—but boxes to be kept ouside room
	Needles—puncture-proof boxes for disposal	
	Syringes—'double-bag' and send for incineration	
Excreta	Dispose into hospital sewage system via bedpan washer/ sterilizer	Dispose into hospital sewage system, via bedpan washer/ sterilizer
	Disposable bedpans/urinals now available in many hospitals, care still needed to avoid contaminating machinery, door handles, etc	Disinfect before taking bedpan/urinal into room, using gloves and polythene covers according to degree of protection
Charts	Should be kept outside room for ease of access	
Laboratory specimens	Should always be safely contained. When double-bag technique applies, use transparent bags and keep form separate from specimen	

Comparative Notes on Isolation Techniques in a Single Bed Sideward
(contd.)

Transport Patients should be taken out of isolation for essential purposes only. Relevant protective clothing must be worn,
and departments involved should be notified in order to
take any necessary action

Cleaning Must be maintained
Surfaces—damp dust with disposable items and discard in
room for source and outside room for protective
isolation
Basin—clean with disposable cloth. Use disinfectant
such as hypochlorite solution to control wet-
medium organisms, e.g. *Pseudomonas* spp.
Floor—separate equipment with launderable or disposable mophead. Wet clean with detergent, and
disinfectant (compatible with mop-head and
detergent)
Clean bucket after use, store dry in room or
separate from other ward equipment

Terminal
cleaning Room—thorough cleaning to include all fittings, with
detergent solution (disinfectant in specified
instances only). Time should be allowed for
thorough drying and ventilation and the room
preferably left for twenty-four hours. Wall-
washing is only needed in special instances or if
heavy soiling has occurred.

Equipment—all removed in appropriate bags for disinfection,
sterilization or incineration as appropriate

13 Problems of Nursing Care for Patients in Isolation —the 'Nursing Process'

All the information contained in the preceding pages should enable nurses and also medical, paramedical and ancillary staff to understand why a particular patient is an infection risk and how this risk can be minimized. This in itself does not constitute total care of such a patient. The 'nursing process' applied to an infected patient's care should attempt to assess not only the potential infection risks—with subsequent planning and implementation to ensure containment—but also what problems and stresses this imposes on the patient, his relatives and friends, other patients and the staff. The nurse has the most contact with a patient and has the best opportunity to assess such problems. She can form plans to alleviate the stresses by avoiding all unnecessary procedures and lightening the sense of genuine 'isolation' the patient may feel. These plans will need frequent evaluation for effectiveness.

Assessment

1. A full *nursing history of the patient* will attempt to discuss the disease/infection with him in order to find out if he understands its implications, mode of transmission and effect upon himself. This will help assess his response to the

disease, acknowledging problems such as fear or distaste, and his acceptance or otherwise of the isolation techniques being applied and the length of time for which they will be applied.

2. The *understanding of family and friends* of the implications of the disease and its treatment will need similar assessment.

3. *Attitudes and fears of other patients* in the ward also need analysis, they too may not understand the disease and fear its implications for them.

4. *Staff understanding* also requires assessment—they will have to take the protective measures required, and will only do so efficiently if they understand the reasons for them and in a helpful and supportive manner to the patient only if they accept this reasoning.

The nurse's powers of drawing inferences, interpreting unspoken or obscurely hinted at problems, and consulting with a range of individuals can be tested severely in this process.

Planning

1. *Determining priorities.* Initially the priority for care of an isolated patient will be to relieve his symptoms and to contain the infection. Once there are plans to deal with these factors, other problems also identified during assessment can be allocated a place and time for action. This will be mostly affected by the patient's attitude, showing the importance he (or others) place upon the problems.

2. *Goals set* to deal with problems must be realistic and precisely stated or they cannot be seen to be achieved. They must also have a definite time limit imposed for the same reason.

3. *The actions to be taken by nursing staff* to achieve

these goals must consider the medical care plan for the patient, and the availability of staff and equipment to care for and support the patient. They must also be discussed with the patient to determine their acceptability within the limitations which this particular form of isolation imposes.

4. *The written plan for the patient's care* must include these actions and their time limits, to check that they are remembered and, hopefully, achieved.

Implementation

1. This must include explanation to the patient of how his illness is being treated, if results are being achieved in terms of his progress, and assurances that no spread of infection is taking place.

2. Friends and family must be given all the necessary information and the opportunity to help the patient and themselves by involvement in care-giving. They can help to find out his worst deprivations and bring in the necessary items, with staff consultation over suitability.

3. The patients on the ward will receive explanation for the isolation of this individual and, if appropriate, receive instruction on the use of protective clothing and will be able to visit him.

4. Explanation to all staff involved with the patient, with demonstration of wearing of clothing, aseptic techniques or methods of disposal of waste food, linen, etc., that they may be reassured for their own safety and be able to make the patient feel that all the techniques are simple and not frightening.

Evaluation

All these actions must be regularly reassessed and altered in tune with the changing situation. Some problems will assume a different priority and proper communication is

Nursing Care Plan for 60-year-old man suffering from Pulmonary Tuberculosis

Problem	Goal	Nursing action	Outcome/Evaluation
Infection—pulmonary Tb	Treat disease and prevent transmission	Drugs as prescribed. Weekly sputum specs. Respiratory isolation	Temperature returns to normal. Cough resolves. Sputum cultures become consistently negative. Able to leave isolation
Extreme apathy, tiredness	Assist to tolerate as temporary	Explain effects of drugs and disease, and that both will ease	Varying levels of acceptance and impatience. Constant encouragement needed
Distressed at isolation, feels cut off from everything	Reduce the sense of isolation	Staff spend more time with patient. Friends encouraged to bring in outside interests. Books, work, radio etc.	Managed to adapt to situation after 2–3 weeks. Took an interest in news and work
Frightened of long illness or death.	Help patient understand modern treatment, and cause of disease	Discussion highlights patient's childhood memories of deaths and sanatorium regimens etc. Re-educated to update knowledge. Discuss progress—temp., sputum results, X-rays etc.	Patient reassured, especially by evidence of lab. reports etc.
Lack of appetite	Stimulate appetite	Consult with dietician. Discover patient's special likes, allow certain food to be brought in to him	Appetite improved slowly. Further explanation (should have been given earlier) of side-effects of drugs

Feels both 'unclean' and unwanted	Acknowledge. Find ways of relieving feelings	Explain protective measures, method of disease transmission. Encourage staff and visitors to talk	Patient gradually appeared to relax. Staff accept having encouraged 'rejected' feeling by lack of time spent in conversation, i.e. administering physical but not social support
Domestic staff neglecting room cleaning	Restore proper cleaning service	Explain disease transmission to domestic staff, and protective measures taken	Cleaning not improved—re-assess and discover staff inadequately trained to use masks etc. Demonstrations. Cleaning standards restored
Patient confused by varying medical and nursing staff use of clothing	Coordinate measures taken by all staff	Meeting of CIO, ICNO, physician, houseman and ward sister—discussion of policy, same endorsed by CIO and physician	Houseman continues to object to clothing policy, but agrees to wear mask at all times and gown when having direct patient contact. Patient reassured
Patient distress at lack of visit from particular relative, fears rejection	Find out reason for absence of relative	Mutual relative asked. Person has been unwell and did not wish to worry patient. Staff get permission to explain to patient	Patient much happier
New member of nursing staff reluctant to help patient at all, appears to avoid entering room	Find out reasons for behaviour, and resolve	Nurse ignorant of need for isolation. Has resented 'extra time' involved in procedures seen as unfair to other patients in the ward. Epidemiology and isolation measures discussed, lack of cross-infection pointed out	Nurse's behaviour altered, much more time spent willingly with patient

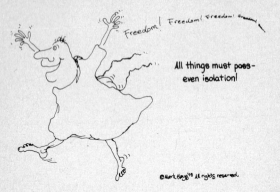

important if the aims of the nursing care plan are to be met. The goals set must therefore be highly specific, with observable criteria related to the patient, not just his condition, and the staff concerned must be able to assess the patient's response objectively. They must also allow time to evaluate the response of friends, relatives and staff. Breakdowns of any sort should be identified, and the reasons for their occurrence analysed to see if there was a way of avoiding them. In a sensibly considered plan of caring for a patient, there should be no reason for failures, but great thought, tact and perseverance are required if all those concerned are to understand and accept the plans involved.

Sterilization Indicators and Tests

AUTOCLAVE CONTROL AND TESTING

Engineers Department	Correct installation with service access. Planned maintenance. (Department of Health and Social Security, Hospital Technical Memorandum No. 10 *Steam Sterilizers.*) Training of the operator.

Autoclave process indicators

Temperature and pressure charts record and present a visual check on the autoclave cycle, steam temperatures and pressures.

Thermometers in the outlet drain and the load simulator register accurate temperatures inside the autoclave; these are displayed on dials on the control panel.

Sterilization process indicators

These are placed in or on each pack to show that it has been through a satisfactory sterilizing process.

Heat/moisture-sensitive tape is plain before autoclaving and develops dark brown stripes or pattern after exposure to steam at sterilizing time/temperature.

Heat-sensitive dyes and inks. These vary in reliability. Colour change.

Heat-sensitive chemicals, e.g. Browne's sterilizer control tubes which contain a chemical which reacts to heat, turning slowly from red (unsterile) to yellow to green. Green indicates satisfactory time/temperature exposure.

Thermolabile plastic melts at a given temperature and flows to a mark on the enclosing tube or sachet. Failure to reach the mark indicates sterilization failure.

Autoclave tests

Thermocouple. This is a temperature recording instrument used to monitor load conditions. One or more sensors (fine probes consisting of two different metals, e.g. copper/constantan) are positioned at test points within the autoclave load, the leads are channelled out through valves in the autoclave wall and linked to a galvanometer, the dial of which gives a constant reading of the temperatures at the test points.

Bowie-Dick test. This is a test to detect any air remaining or leaking into a high vacuum autoclave during the cycle. Procedure see Fig. 48. It is not a suitable test for any other type of autoclave.

Air leak test. This is a method of detecting air leaking into the chamber through a faulty valve or door seal. The autoclave is closed, the vacuum drawn on manual control, and the valves then closed to isolate the chamber. The vacuum should be maintained; a decrease in vacuum of more than 10 mm Hg during 10 minutes holding time indicates an air leak and the machine requires servicing by an engineer before use. Test for high vacuum autoclaves only.

Huckaback towels 3ft x 2ft (B.S. 1781 TL5)
washed and aired stack
10 to 11 in. high

Centre of stack   a St Andrew's cross of 3M
brand autoclave tape No. 1222
on a sheet of paper (NOT waxed)
or a sheet of 3M No. 1222

Enclose towels   in a standard pack wrap
or 'sterilizing box'
in a firm pack

Test pack ONLY   is placed in the autoclave
on the bottom shelf

Normal autoclave cycle is run

SATISFACTORY   UNSATISFACTORY

Fig. 48. The Bowie-Dick autoclave test.

Biological testing. Heat resistant spores, usually of *Bacillus stearothermophilus,* are placed in test packs in a normal load, they are then sent to the laboratory for culture which takes up to five days. Only an efficient autoclave will kill these spores. This method of testing is infrequently used for routine purposes, largely because of the time factor.

HOT AIR OVEN TESTS AND INDICATORS

Temperature charts record the time cycle and the temperature within the oven, but not within the load.

Thermocouple testing is essential in order to set the correct time cycle.

Heat-sensitive chemicals or tape are used to indicate by colour change that an item has been through a dry heat sterilizing process. Foil sealing caps often carrying a colour change indicator, a wide range is available, e.g. blue to pink, red to gold.

GAMMA IRRADIATION STERILIZATION INDICATOR

The most commonly used indicator is a small, circular, adhesive disc which changes in colour from yellow to red.

ETHYLENE OXIDE STERILIZATION INDICATOR

Green gas-sensitive tape turns from deep to pale green after exposure to ethylene oxide gas. Care must be taken not to leave an unsterile load in the sterilizer as even traces of the gas will complete the colour change in about 24 hours.

A chemical solution enclosed in a sachet turns from yellow to purple after exposure to ethylene oxide gas. The time taken to effect the change depends on the temperature.

Biological testing. *Bacillus subtilis (globigii)* spores are used.

Appendix II

Environmental Sampling Methods

Fluids Collect with a sterile syringe and needle, Transfer into a sterile laboratory container.

Surfaces Use a sterile swab, e.g. throat swab. Moisten with sterile broth or sterile distilled water for dry surfaces. Rotate the swab whilst rubbing it lightly and evenly over the surface.

Fabrics (a) Contact plates. Fabric is pressed lightly on to the surface of an agar plate. Avoid contamination from hands by wearing a disposable polythene glove or 'bunching up' the fabric.

(b) Sweep plates. An area of fabric 30–60 cm is stretched and an inverted agar plate swept up and down it 10 times with the plate edges in contact with the fabric.

Tubing Bacteriologists often prefer to sample tubing in the laboratory where it can be sectioned. Sterile broth is injected at one end, allowed to flow slowly through the tubing, and is collected into a sterile laboratory container at the other end. Care must be taken to avoid contamination from the outside of the tubing ends.

Air (a) Flow is observed by tracing smoke generated by, e.g. titanium tetrachloride which forms dense white smoke when in contact with atmospheric moisture.

(b) Volume and direction are measured with a vane anemometer.

(*c*) Humidity is measured with an hygrometer or calculated from wet and dry bulb thermometer readings.

(*d*) Cleanliness is measured by counting bacteria collected by: (*i*) *settle plates.* Agar plates are exposed for a specified time (usually 15 minutes). Bacteria collected on the surface are identified and counted. (*ii*) *Air sampling machines,* e.g. Bourdillon slit sampler which draws air at the rate of 1 ft^3 per minute, through a narrow slit on to the surface of an agar plate 2 mm below. The plate rests on a small turntable which completes its revolution in a fixed time, for example 5 minutes. The slit equals the radius of the plate. Using such equipment, an accurate estimate of the numbers of bacteria in a room can be made.

IN-USE TESTING OF DISINFECTANTS

Kelsey and Maurer (1974) describe a practical method of sampling and assessing the efficiency of disinfectant solutions which are actually in use in a working situation, e.g. in a urinal disinfection tank or a floor scrubbing machine reservoir. 1 ml of disinfectant solution in use is collected with a sterile pipette and added to 9 ml of diluent in a sterile container. The diluent is selected according to the disinfectant and the site of use, and is supplied by the bacteriology laboratory. The container is sent straight back to the laboratory for processing. Two agar plates are inoculated. One is incubated at 37°C for three days, the other at room temperature for seven days. The plates are then examined and the results reported.

If bacteria are grown the disinfectant fails the test, i.e. is failing to kill bacteria in the situation and in the strength at which it is in use.

Chemical disinfection is unreliable and many hospitals therefore have a routine in-use testing programme.

'SEE FOR YOURSELF'—SUGGESTIONS FOR EXPERIMENTS IN CONJUNCTION WITH LABORATORIES AND SCHOOLS OF NURSING

Respiratory tract bacteria
1. Cough on to an agar plate held about 10 cm from the mouth.
2. Compare the telephone mouthpiece of a ward and a public telephone (moistened swab).
3. Swab an oxygen or anaesthetic mask immediately after use.
4. Swab the inside of a used toothmug.

Skin bacteria
1. Swab a bath 'tide line', clean the bath and swab again. Compare the results.
2. A used communal towel contact plate.
3. Dirty, washed but wet, then well dried hands. In each situation make fingerprints on an agar plate by rolling the tip of each finger in turn lightly on the surface of a separate area of the plate (see Chapter 11).
4. Settle plate exposed in a ward during bedmaking, place on the floor by the end of a bed, expose for 15 minutes. Compare with a plate exposed when the ward is quiet.

Intestinal bacteria, wet medium bacteria
1. Swab under the rim of a bedpan.
2. The next sheet of toilet paper. Contact plate.
3. Sample of flower water.
4. Kitchen sink cloth. Contact plate.

5. Floor cloth or mop. Contact plate.
6. Drain trap. Sample as far down the drain as can be reached with a throat swab.

Multiplication Factors

Multiplication factor	Prefix	Symbol
$1\,000\,000\,000\,000 = 10^{12}$	tera	T
$1\,000\,000\,000 = 10^{9}$	giga	G
$1\,000\,000 = 10^{6}$	mega	M
$1\,000 = 10^{3}$	kilo	k
$100 = 10^{2}$	hecto	h
$10 = 10^{1}$	deca	da
$0.1 = 10^{-1}$	deci	d
$0.01 = 10^{-2}$	centi	c
$0.001 = 10^{-3}$	milli	m
$0.000\,001 = 10^{-6}$	micro	μ
$0.000\,000\,001 = 10^{-9}$	nano	n
$0.000\,000\,000\,001 = 10^{-12}$	pico	p
$0.000\,000\,000\,000\,001 = 10^{-15}$	femto	f
$0.000\,000\,000\,000\,000\,001 = 10^{-18}$	atto	a

Equivalents

$$m\mu = nm = \text{nanometre } (10^{-9})$$
$$\mu = \mu m = \text{micrometre } (10^{-6})$$

Length:

1 foot = 0.305 metres
3 feet = 0.915 metres

Weight:

2.205 pounds = 1000 grams = 1 kilogram

Energy:

1 calorie = 4.2 joules (J)

Capacity:

1 pint = 0.568 litres

Temperature:

Fahrenheit (F) minus 32 multiplied by 5/9 = C
Celsius (C) multiplied by 9/5 plus 32 = F

$<$ = less than
$>$ = greater than

Selected Further Reading

HISTORY BOOKS

Baldry, P.E. (1976) *The Battle against Bacteria. A History of the Development of Antibacterial Drugs for the General Reader*, 2nd ed. London: Cambridge University Press.

Cuny, H. (1965) *Louis Pasteur: The Man and his Theories*, Translated by Patrick Evans. London: Souvenir Press.

Guthrie, Douglas (1949) *Lord Lister. His Life and Doctrine*. Edinburgh: Livingstone.

Ludovici, L.J. (1958) *The World of the Infinitely Small*. London: Dent.

Manson-Bahr, Sir Phillip (1962) *Patrick Manson—The Father of Tropical Medicine*. London: Thomas Nelson.

Maurois, A. (1963) *The Life of Alexander Fleming*. Harmondsworth: Penguin.

Parish, H.J. (1968) *Victory with Vaccine*. Edinburgh: Livingstone.

Wilson, J.R. (1963) *Margin of Safety. The Story of Poliomyelitis Vaccine*. London: Collins.

MICROBIOLOGY BOOKS

Christie, A.B. (1980) *Infectious Diseases*. London: Churchill Livingstone.

Frobisher, M. & others (1969) *Microbiology for Nurses*, 11th ed. Philadelphia: Saunders.

Garrod, L.P., Lambert, H.P. & O'Grady, F. (1973) *Antibiotics and Chemotherapy*, 4th ed. Edinburgh: Livingstone.

Gillies, R.R. & Dodds, T.C. (1976) *Bacteriology Illus-trated*, 4th ed. Edinburgh: Livingstone.

Halliday, W.J. (1971) *Glossary of Immunological Terms*. London: Butterworths.

Olds, R.J. (1975) *A Colour Atlas of Microbiology*. London: Wolfe Medical.

Ross, P.W. (1979) *Clinical Bacteriology*. London: Churchill Livingstone.

Stokes, J. (1978) *Clinical Bacteriology*. London: Edward Arnold.

Tighe, J.R. (1972) *Pathology*, 3rd ed. London: Baillière Tindall.

Timbury, M.C. (1977) *Notes on Medical Virology*. Edin-burgh: Livingstone.

Turk, D.C. & Porter, I.A. (1978) *A Short Textbook of Medical Microbiology*. London: Hodder & Stoughton.

Weir, D.M. (1977) *Immunology*. London: Churchill Livingstone.

Advanced

Cruickshank, R. (1972/1975) *Medical Microbiology*, Vols. I & II, 12th ed. Edinburgh: Livingstone.

Jawetz, E. *et al.* (1976) *Review of Medical Microbiology*, 12th ed. California: Lange.

Rhodes, A.J. & Van Rooyen, C.E. (1962) *Textbooks of Virology*. Baltimore: Williams & Wilkins.

Sykes, G. (1975) *Disinfection and Sterilization*, 2nd ed. London: Chapman & Hall.

Topley & Wilson. Principles of bacteriology and im-munology. London: Arnold.

APPLIED MICROBIOLOGY BOOKS

Benenson, A.S. (1975) *Control of Communicable Diseases in Man*, 12th ed. American Public Health Association.

Emmerson, A.M. & Jenner, E.A. (1978) *Infection Control Manual*. Islington District of the Camden and Islington Area Health Authority (Teaching): London.

Gibson, G.L. (1974) *Infection in Hospitals. A Code of Practice,* 2nd ed. Edinburgh and London: Churchill Livingstone.

Lowbury, E.J.L. *et al.* (1975) *Control of Hospital Infection.* London: Chapman & Hall.

Maurer, I.M. (1978) *Hospital Hygiene,* 2nd ed. London: Edward Arnold.

Parry, W.H. (1973) *Communicable Diseases. An Epidemiological Approach,* 2nd ed. London: English Universities Press.

Smillie, W.G. & Kilbourne, E.D. (1963) *Preventive Medicine and Public Health.* London: Macmillan.

US Department of Health, Education and Welfare (1975) *Isolation Techniques for Use in Hospitals,* 2nd ed. Public Health Services.

REPORTS AND ARTICLES

Thousands of reports and articles, in English and other languages, are published every year. Regular reading of journals such as *The Nursing Times, The Nursing Mirror,* and the *International Nursing Review* will introduce topics of current concern and interest; some other journals and official bodies which regularly publish important original reports and articles on microbiological topics are listed below. All nurses, in particular those concerned with teaching or infection control should have access to these journals:

British Medical Journal
Journal of Clinical Pathology
Journal of Hospital Infections
Journal of Hygiene
Journal of Infection
Journal of Infection Control Nursing
Journal of Medical Microbiology
Lancet
Sterile World (publishes the proceedings of the Central Sterilizing Club)

Department of Health and Social Security, and *The Scottish Home and Health Department*

A list of publications is available from HMSO Memoranda to National Health Service Hospitals, e.g. HM(69) 'Preservation of sterility in ophthalmic preparations used in hospitals.'

King Edward's Hospital Fund for London

Also have a reference Library and advisory Hospital Centre in London.

The Medical Research Council

E.g. Aseptic methods in the operating suite. A report by the sub-committee on aseptic methods in operating theatres of the Committee on Hospital Infection (1968).

Lancet **i,** 705, 763, 831.

Nuffield Provincial Hospitals Trust

E.g. *Central Sterile Supply. Principles and Practice* (1963) Oxford University Press.

Public Health Laboratory Service

The weekly Communicable Disease Reports include brief epidemiological studies as well as national statistics.

World Health Organization

WHO Chronicle. A monthly record of WHO assisted health activities for the medical and public health professions.

Bulletin of the WHO. Technical articles by physicians and scientists engaged in public health work.

World Health. An illustrated magazine for the general public. Also technical reports and statistics.

Laboratory aspects of the prevention and control of hospital-acquired infection (1979).

Index